New Mind

New Body

The Inner Makeover
for a New You

By

Gregory Brown, MD

Board Certified Psychiatrist

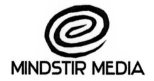

Rave Reviews for New Mind New Body

Dr. Greg has written the book I have been seeking for decades. If you have issues with weight, this is the definitive source for how to address them effectively. Read it today--it will change your life.

--Wendy Long

Dr. Brown invites us to take a new approach in the journey of weight loss. This book acts as a guide through a very real self-inventory in addition to providing practical strategies with the goal of providing long term success.

- Alison Netski, M.D., Assistant Professor of Psychiatry, University of Nevada School of Medicine

I wanted to let you know that after reading your book and talking to you, I started "taking steps" and have lost 2 dress sizes and FEEL GREAT!!! I am making great food choices. I mentally changed "gym" to "spa" (which I go to almost daily now and do between 6K-10K steps) and the word "diet" to the phrase "I am taking steps towards health". It's because of you! Your book and program has made a huge difference to me. Thank you so much!

--Ann McIndoo, Author

Dr. Brown's natural ability to resonate with people and motivate them to institute positive change has been an inspiration to me. His mentorship has helped me in my own development.

--*Faisal Suba, M.D.*

Dr. Brown's guidance over the years has provided me with clarity into who I am and what I wish to accomplish. He has a remarkable talent in helping others navigate through the complex nature of life situations.

--*Syed K. Abubaker, M.D.*

This book is an excellent introduction to the psychology of eating, with material to satisfy both beginners and experts. It is deftly written, clear yet detailed, and I heartily recommend it to anyone interested in the subject.

-- *Michael R. Madow, M.D., Fellow of the American Psychiatric Association*

Dedication

I dedicate this information to everyone who has ever struggled to lose pounds only to become lost in the struggle. My dream is that your journey can be made clearer and successful.

Acknowledgements

I would first like to express my appreciation and gratitude to my wife, Alicia, who has always supported new ventures, new learning, and new experience. She has been an encouragement and support whether she was aware of it or not.

So many deserve thanks for their critical roles in helping this project come to fruition: the team at Speaking Empire Dave VanHoose, Dustin Matthews, Caroline Mehle and Anthony Ellis, who helped build this dream from an idea into reality; Imran Rahman at Rahman Media, and his team who supported and created the online content; Ann McIndoo, my Author's Coach, who helped get this book out of my head.

Special thanks to colleagues and friends who provided feedback and ideas throughout the process.

Contents

Introduction

You are probably wondering why you should even consider trying this program. After all, you have probably tried a series of short-term diets only to see the weight lost return with a few extra pounds; in short: the diet yo-yo. I lived through that discouraging pattern and discovered a way out of it. And if I can do it, I know you can too.

Who am I? I am a psychiatrist who has evaluated hundreds of patients considering gastric bypass surgery and Lap-Band placement surgery. I have had the opportunity to hear and understand their stories. I bring the knowledge and skill set of a physician to understand the problem of continuing weight difficulties and problems. Perhaps you have spoken to your doctor about weight loss, and may believe my credentials are not enough.

The real reason you might choose to read this book is my own personal lifelong challenges with weight control and answers that I have discovered over the course of time.

It is stunning to me, in retrospect, to recall that throughout the entirety of medical school, I had a total of two hours of lecture time devoted to diet, food and appropriate food choices in a curriculum that lasted four years. This was followed by four years of residency and an additional year of fellowship, which never raised the topic, in spite of recommending weight loss to many patients during that timeframe.

My weight journey began in high school when I started gaining weight and did not have a good way of stopping it. Up-and-down diets, trying everything from low-fat to low-carb to half portions to exercise all worked briefly, but soon followed weight gain beyond the amount lost.

In approximately 2011, I hit my weight pinnacle of 248 pounds after stepping off a wonderful cruise that my wife and I enjoyed in Alaska. When I got home and weighed myself, I was horrified, disgusted, and absolutely fed up with myself in pretty much every way that I could imagine.

I went on a halfhearted low-carb diet at that point and dropped a few pounds, then got disgusted with that and stopped, followed by a half-portion diet, which I will discuss later, and then got completely stuck. I knew that I would not undergo a surgical procedure for this problem, and I knew that I would not take any form of medication to lose weight either.

In one of those shower insights I realized, "You are a psychiatrist. If anyone can figure this out, it is you, so get to it!"

First, I extensively searched for books and other materials with the focus on the actual path of what was needed to psychologically change in order to successfully lose weight, and I found exceptionally little as a guide or a help in this entire process. As I began to work through layers and issues and explore different parts of myself that led me down a successful path of weight loss, I began to understand that this was a bigger picture than a simple set of behavioral challenges.

One insight that came to me was from a rather archaic psychoanalytic term called "overdetermination" or "overdetermined symptoms." Once I was able to see weight challenges as being an overdetermined symptom, this opened a series of doors that allowed me to change the various pieces of myself using a series of techniques I will share.

I will discuss overdetermination in a later chapter, but it is one of the keys to understanding why weight is such a big challenge over a lifetime. I was able to successfully lose sixty pounds and astound my family physician by lowering my blood cholesterol by over forty points in the process. I used a specific diet, but the change was that the diet became a comfortable lifestyle rather than an obstacle to fight against.

One metaphor I envisioned that helped put this entire principal into a larger picture is the metaphor of a string a pearls in which each episode of eating or desiring food or picking food or choosing food or putting it in your mouth matches a pattern that you have developed over the course of a lifetime. That pattern is represented by the shape of an energetic string created by life experience. You place each food-related experience onto this vibrant string, provided they match the shape of the string. Chips fit on the string when you feel upset, celery sticks, not so much.

If you had a choice of a good food or a bad food, you are going to pick the food that matches your experience, or your string, rather than picking something that would suit your new health goals.

Until you identify the characteristics of your string, you will continue to automatically put pearls on that string no matter how unhealthy or unreasonable they are. This drives the unconscious desire for foods and particular food groups that are likely the opposite of your consciously stated goal of weight loss.

The awesome piece of information is that there are a series of techniques that you can use after you have identified the string, or the core of the string, to begin breaking up the pearls and reshape the string to allow you to naturally eat more healthily without feeling deprived and without feeling as if you are missing something, which changes the entire emotional complex of eating into a more healthy endeavor.

I will be including various stories from patients and others interwoven throughout the book. Because my field requires an exceptionally high degree of confidentiality, there will be no identifying information presented about these individuals. Everything irrelevant to the point will be disguised in every measure – gender, job, age – however, the central point of each particular story will be clear and representative of that individual's life experiences.

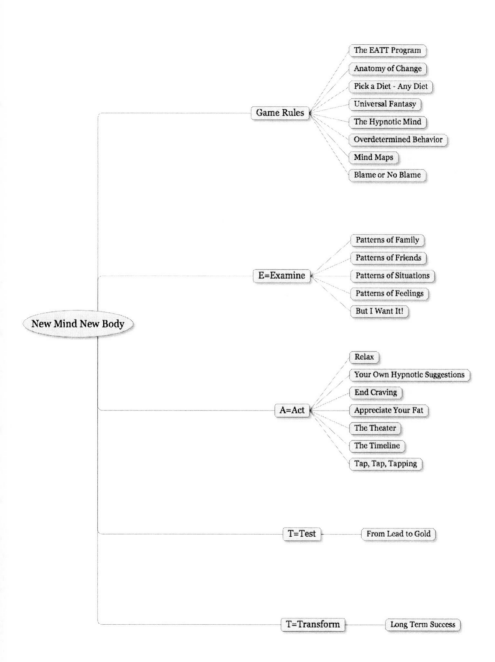

DISCLAIMER

The materials and activities in this book and the accompanying support book will contain evocative techniques to bring up information and patterns from the past. This should be quite safe for the average adult; however, if you are already engaged in therapy, if you have a diagnosis of a psychiatric disorder, please use this book with the aid of a trained professional therapist to help you through the difficult points, as inadvertently some memories or information could come into awareness that could best be dealt with in a formal psycho-therapeutic relationship. Dr. Brown is providing information, not treatment.

Likewise, if information comes up that is overwhelming in the course of the book, please do seek professional guidance to deal with those painful memories should the techniques provided here not fully resolve them in as painless a manner as possible.

Weight loss is a journey with many complicated facets. Although these techniques are based upon clear, well-founded principles, no guarantee is made regarding your specific weight loss goals.

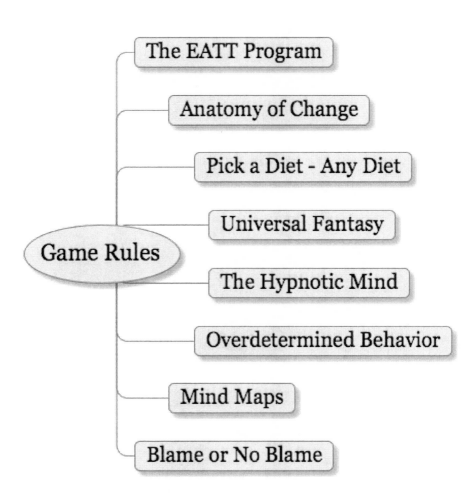

The EATT Program

Anatomy of Change

Pick a Diet - Any Diet

Universal Fantasy

Game Rules

The Hypnotic Mind

Overdetermined Behavior

Mind Maps

Blame or No Blame

Chapter One

Game Rules: The EATT Program

You Are the Hero of This Journey

The process of successful and ongoing weight loss does require internal change, and this internal change is very well represented by the journey of the hero. That is a painful sentence to start a book with. Re-read it. Everyone hates change. It is part of our internal makeup, because not changing seems to be so much more comfortable. But change is something we have all successfully negotiated before.

Think back to second grade. At the end of that year, spelling, writing, addition and subtraction were all new skills that were mastered; a journey of knowledge and learning that made the little grade school student into a hero. Now those skills are second nature. But learning the rudiments of math and language were the challenges of the year, and successful completion changed the mind and the concepts of that young person. This is the journey of the hero.

Joseph Campbell, the famous comparative mythologist, described this journey of the hero as a four-stage process beginning with the call to adventure. This was followed by the tests of guardians to assess resolve. The third phase would test the hero's core weakness. When the hero then was successful in the fourth and final phase, the return to the world to share the triumph grounded the growth in consciousness.

This outer journey that Campbell talks about is actually representative of an inner journey of change. Had the hero failed to heed the call, they would have never engaged on the journey, or had they been unable to negotiate that key point of inner change, they would have failed in the journey and returned back without successfully completing the task. The essential failure in the cycle, though, is failing to transform through the process of the journey,. for the hero emerges as a different person than the one who began the journey.

It is easy to see this kind of change in cinema, as an example in movies, such as *Lord of the Rings* or *Star Wars*, in which the main character ends the story as a transformed person. Contrast this with some of the early action movies, such as the James Bond adventures. The Bond stories are interesting and full of action, but they do not represent a change in Bond's character because at the end of each movie, he is essentially the same person.

The first phase of the hero's journey is accepting the call to adventure. This is exactly where you stand now as you begin opening this book and start to read its very pages. You can reject the call and put the book back on the shelf or accept the call and begin this process of inner change.

What I can assure you is if you fail to allow process to promote personal transformation, you will equally fail at creating a new pattern of eating that could last for you.

Getting Off the Psychological Couch

It may or may not be necessary to engage in substantial physical exercise in order to lose weight, but that is not the purpose of this book. We are going to be looking at doing mental exercise and emotional exercise, which are equally important for personal change.

The book is designed in a linear fashion. Beware, jumping to a final chapter that looks interesting may prove difficult to understand without foundation of the earlier material. I would encourage you to follow this process through the book in the same way that you will be following an interior journey of change.

There is a series of exercises - titled "experiences" - throughout the book. We all hate the word "exercise" so I have avoided that term! These experiences can all be completed without leaving the chair.

The other step, in the beginning, is to suspend disbelief. Some of the experiences may seem as if they do not apply, but play along and have fun, complete the process. Later, you can look back and see how successful or how unsuccessful each technique was.

Some of the exercises later in the book may feel more helpful than others, and there is some overlap in their effectiveness, so choose those that are most successful after experiencing them all.

Brutal Self-Honesty

How many of us have ever sat down and played a game of solitaire with a deck of cards and run out of options? How many reshuffle the cards or turn a few over just to successfully finish the game? That is perfectly fine in solitaire, but it will absolutely fail for long-term personal change.

We must obtain data honestly and clearly. First, we are going to require honesty in weight, so get rid of that old scale that has a shot spring in it that underweighs the doctor's scale by at least ten pounds, and go purchase a real scale that has an ability to calculate BMI as well as weight to ensure accurate information day after day.

Second, start a food diary, which I will discuss later, but complete it with the willingness to be entirely honest. To alter calorie intake, it is necessary to know the number of calories actually consumed.

Third, and most important for this journey, is complete honesty in terms of self-reflection. There may be aspects of us that are uncomfortable or that we do not want to approach because eating is a complicated behavior that has been modified since very early childhood, sometimes by experiences that were not entirely pleasant. These experiences cannot hurt you any longer; however, we often like to avoid them.

Ten Free Behavioral Tips

I am going to include ten behavioral clues and tips throughout the book, randomly through chapters, and I can assure you that if you were to follow all ten of these tips for an extended period of time, you could successfully lose weight even by ignoring everything else in the book; however, I can equally promise you that you will fail if you attempt this.

The reason failure is eminent with following simple behavior changes is the same reason that every diet in the past failed. Willpower is required to follow both behavioral changes and dietary changes, and willpower always fails for creating long-term change. The reason willpower will always fail will be discussed in the chapter on the hypnotic mind.

The journey of the EATT Program teaches that not only are you what you eat, but, in fact, you eat what you are. As you become a new person, that which you eat will change. The journey is as important as the outcome, so savor the journey rather than rushing to outcome.

The EATT Program is a program designed to help with eating more consciously so that food nourishes your body, mind and spirit.

"E" stands for "Examine," which we will accomplish using exercises to bring up issues, people, emotions and places from the past, and explore how that affects eating behavior today. We will typically use mind maps, or some variant of mind maps, to compile the different pieces in one clumping of understanding, and we will discuss that process later in the book as well. This is the idea of identifying the characteristics of the string on which your food pearls lie.

"A" is to "Act," which we will accomplish by utilizing the experiences later in the book to neutralize cravings, to reduce the emotional impact of various past experiences on present eating. This will deconstruct the string upon which the food pearls lie and to allow new realities of food choice.

"T" is to "Test." After the Action, explore how successful the result has been. If useful, it is a new self-intervention. If not, return to "Examine" and repeat.

The final "T" is the "Transformation" that naturally follows from the first three steps. This represents a new shape of string for a new grouping of food related pearls. Certainly do not forget to celebrate at this point as well.

The last step of Campbell's hero's journey is a return to the world. Individuals who simply go off and make changes but never return back to the world tend to never ground them in a way that makes them permanent.

You have all probably met individuals who meditate all the time and get very airy and spacey and seem to lack realistic contact with the world. This is not the goal of your journey.

After personal transformation occurs, bring it back to

the world and ground it by documenting the inner growth that has occurred. The last experience of the book will be the writing of the story of your hero's journey which will iron this entire process down very effectively.

Chapter Two

The Anatomy of Change

One of the most amazing things that I have had the opportunity to experience as a psychiatrist in clinical practice is hearing the stories of people who have successfully made giant changes in their lives and compare those to the stories of people who have not. The most interesting question to me is, what is different between those stories and why?

Sally was a female who had engaged in long-term alcohol use to the extent that her life was significantly impacted and she was on the brink of becoming deathly ill with liver disease. She had stopped drinking altogether, from a particular life event forward.

She shared that the joy of becoming a grandmother led to the intense realization that if she did not change her life and change her behavior that she would not have the chance of seeing her granddaughter graduate from college. At the time I met Sally, her granddaughter was already in high school.

It was that single event that was so deeply meaningful to her in a personal way that led her to stop a behavior that literally hundreds of people had told her for decades was deleterious to her health.

Another example of this was Cornelia who had engaged in smoking tobacco for a period of decades at a consumption of over six packs per day. She sought out physicians who would not confront her about tobacco use because she knew it was the best way to relax. She realized the health problems associated with the behavior, but chose to accept those risks and engage in smoking anyway. This continued up until the point at which a loved one passed away from lung cancer in her arms. Starting that day, she never smoked another cigarette.

Again, another example of a profound life situation which caused immediate, permanent, lasting change and it did so by changing the values that each of these individuals held towards a behavior which had been out of control. It also occurred in the context of a deep level of inner meaning undergoing dramatic transformation.

Both of these individuals had been told by family, friends, and doctors, probably for decades, that what they were doing was unhealthy. None of that information changed their behavior because it did not impact anything beyond their conscious awareness. It was only a piece of knowledge and a request which failed to affect their perception of reality.

For them, smoking and drinking were the pearls on their string, and they were not willing to change the string or remove the pearls until a major life event happened. At which point, the string transformed and the pearls dropped off of their own accord.

Transformation: From Live to Eat to Eat to Live

One of the things that I have noticed when speaking with individuals who are either overweight or at normal weight is that they value eating in a very different manner in life.
People who tend to be at a normal weight for their body stature will often say things such as, "I don't want to take the time to eat. Eating is a chore for me," or "I have to make an effort to go find something to eat because it is not at the top of my list of things to do."

In contrast, people who tend to be overweight plan their day around eating, so meals will be one of the primary things that they focus upon, and other things happen to fall between meals. This is a clue in terms of a behavioral schema of what is important in life, and we want to make a transformation in the context of this journey so that eating becomes a choice, not a compelled behavior.

EXPERIENCE #1: WHY NOW?

Take out a piece of paper. Remember, I promised that you have to get off of the psychological couch and do something, so get the paper, and write down on this paper a list of every reason that comes to your mind right now as you sit here of why you wish to lose weight. Take ten minutes. Make the list as long as you possibly can and do not look ahead in this explanation until you have completed the list in its entirety.

Feel free to put the first few on the lines included here or use the form in the section labeled "Chapter Two" in the Action Book.

1. _____

_____

2. _____

_____

3. _____

_____

4. _____

_____

5. _____

_____

After you have completed the list, take a large red pen and mark through any reason that you have come up with that takes the form of other people telling you something. For example, if one of the reasons is *my doctor told me to lose weight*, mark through that with a red pen. If it is *my spouse told me to lose weight* or *my children think I should lose weight* or *my coworkers wish I would lose weight* or *people keep putting diet drinks in front of me instead of the regular Coke*, all of those reasons get a red line. The only reason that does not get a red line is some variant of *it is a core desire for me at this time to lose weight*.

Rewrite all of those other reasons that have red lines through them in this new format now. For example, change *my kids want me to lose weight* into *it is my core desire to see my children graduate from college and losing weight will help me to become healthy enough to do that*. In making the rewrite of the reasons marked out in red, you assume ownership of the reason for weight loss rather than placing responsibility on others.

If the ownership is on other people for the *why now* question, you are destined to fail. Remember, honesty.

If you cannot come up with a reason for yourself to proceed on this journey, then realize you have declined the opportunity to continue, at least for now. You are refusing the call to be the hero, and that is perfectly acceptable because this time may not be your time to start. Close the book, put it on the shelf, and when you are ready to start this process, you can start back on this very exercise, and at the point you actually create some compelling "I" statements that will support your journey, then, and only then, move forward.

BEHAVIOR TIP #1: CHEW ANYTHING YOU EAT TWENTY TIMES

There are several behavioral tips which are interlinked with one another over the course of this book, many of which are designed to slow down the eating process. The primary biological reason for slowing food intake is that it requires approximately twenty to thirty minutes for your stomach to begin registering a sensation of being full or satisfied to your brain.

One way to slow down our eating process is to chew food more times than we are accustomed to. We tend to live in a fast-food culture where people have a fifteen-minute lunch; they grab something as large as they can, then chew it as fast as possible, and wolf it down without ever enjoying the taste. So, the first step in slowing down the eating process is to chew everything twenty times. If soup is on the menu and it is chunky, chew it twenty times. If the soup is watery, savor the flavor for double the time and use that as an effective substitution for what is essentially a liquid.

Of Addictions and Rewards

Many people characterize the process of overeating under a concept or a model of addiction, and in fact we hear the words "food addiction" tossed around quite freely in social settings. There is nothing necessarily wrong with this term, but I object to it because of the public conception that if we are addicted to something, we no longer have any control over it or behavior surrounding it. If you have a different notion of addiction in your head, awesome, keep it.

The general truths are that addictions of any sort to any type of substance or behavior relate to activation of the reward circuitry of the brain, typically parts of the dopamine system, and because the dopamine system mediates behavior and experiences that we tend to find pleasurable, continued activation of this system relates in behavior that we see as behaviorally addicting.

However, there is another part of the brain that is deeply tied to any form of behavior, and that is the association network. The association network contains all of the meaning structures that we associate with everything we do.

In order for a behavior to become addicting and attach to the dopaminergic circuit and in order for these to become connected to one another, there has to be some kind of meaning in the association cortex that mediates the pleasure and gives it context.

The individuals whom I discussed at the beginning of this chapter were addicted to the various substances, and if we looked at it from a purely genetic and a purely biological viewpoint, these people could never have stopped using the substance, ever, under any circumstances, because the biology would have suggested they could have remained and would have remained addicted forever.

The glimmer of hope in this biological model of addiction is that the genetic component of the association network where we keep the meanings of our life is zero. The genetics may make us susceptible to being addicted to alcohol or to eating or to other kinds of behavior, but we have almost complete control over how we develop meaning about things.

The key neurological dictum is that neurons that wire together, fire together, and neurons that fire together, wire together. That is how these circuits are created.

If we create a new meaning in life just like Sally and Cornelia at the beginning of the chapter, we disconnect the addictive behavior from the reward circuity in a single act. This is the hope for each of us as we progress down this hero's journey. To disconnect the addictive portion of eating from the reward circuitry that supports it by changing the meaning associated with the eating behavior.

Again, genetic influences do affect the actual reward circuitry, and it may make it very easy for a particular individual to become "addicted" to something, but our layer of choice lies into what we connect to this reward circuitry through the association network.

Chapter Three

Pick a Diet – Any Diet

This plan is designed to work with any diet that consistently followed. It supports any of the mainstream diets on the market whether they involve an overall reduction in calories, an overall reduction in fat, or an overall reduction in carbohydrates.

This chapter will, however, help you choose the diet that would be most appropriate.

Three Food Groups

There exist three types of nutritional content in food [beyond vitamins].

• Carbohydrates, which consist of sugar, starches (potatoes, pasta, bread and wheat), and fiber.

• Protein, which consists of meat, tofu, fish, chicken, pork, and seafood.
• Fat.

The bad news in this story is that we all have a genetic purpose, and that is, our genes will tell us to store fat whenever possible. The reason for this, in all likelihood, is that millennia ago when food ran short, people who did not store fat effectively died of starvation. The people who survived passed on the genes which promoted fat storage in the body rather than fat breakdown in the body.

Over the course of millennia, genes promoting fat storage would have been selected out as being the most likely for each of us to receive at the time of our birth. This does not indicate that it is impossible to lose weight, however, as we can alter genetic expression and metabolism based upon our particular diet.

Cut Calories and One, and Only One, Other Thing

This leaves the choice as being relatively straightforward in theory. The body requires protein in order to maintain muscle mass, so protein is not a safe option on the list of things to cut. Therefore, there are only two choices left.

You can either cut carbohydrates, i.e., sugar, or you can cut fat. If you attempt to cut both, I have seen patients whose bodies have resisted weight loss with an amazing tenacity. I suspect this drastic reduction put the body into a starvation mode such that it does everything possible to prevent weight loss.

There is an entirely different metabolic pathway involved depending on the choice. If we choose to cut fats from our diet, then we will continue in a sugar-burning type of metabolism. The body will burn sugar as its primary fuel source and any excess sugar at the end of the day that is not utilized will be transformed into fat for storage, basically storing energy for when it may later be needed.

If, on the other hand, you reduce carbohydrates markedly from your diet but continue to consume fat, your body will adapt into a new metabolic pattern called ketosis in which fat and cholesterol become primary fuel sources for energy. The conversion between a sugar-based diet and a fat- and protein-based diet takes approximately two weeks to fully accomplish, which is why some who attempt low-carb diets feel as if they have the flu for the first ten to fourteen days. This misery typically resolves when the body has fully switched to a ketosis-based metabolism, at which point energy levels throughout the day tend to be more constant.

There are two key messages from this particular point. First, it is necessary to pick one or the other. It is not possible to switch from low-fat diet bars to low-carb diet bars and go back and forth indiscriminately because the body cannot keep up with the metabolic changes that are involved in doing this day by day. So pick one and stick with it.

The second issue is that this is a long-term choice, so find a particular set of foods that you will be comfortable eating, with little sense of deprivation.

I indicated earlier that we physicians get about two hours of education in diet in all of the many years we go to school, but nevertheless, it is necessary to check with your doctor to see if you have any particular overriding health needs that would make one diet versus another preferable for your health.

The other thing to check with your doctor about is medications or conditions you have that may make weight loss more of a challenge, to evaluate whether alternatives are possible.

Top Eight Medications that Cause Weight Gain

I will start this section with a brief caveat, and that is if you are on one or more of these medications, do not stop taking until you have spoken with your doctor about it to see if there is a suitable alternative. It may be that some of these medications cause weight gain, but it also may be that it is necessary for other aspects of health. If so, negotiate with your doctor over time, but do not abruptly stop it because of this potential side effect.

I can give you an example of William, a gentleman whom I treated for an extended period of time with antipsychotic medications. These medications allowed him to function in a professional work setting, and in absence of these medications, he would have been homebound.

He made the choice to continue taking the medication even though it caused him a fifty-pound weight gain over the course of approximately six months. There were no reasonable alternatives for him in terms of treatment, and he decided that he would actively diet and exercise, and when I saw him about three months later, he lost most of that weight by exercising daily and eating only salads and a bit of protein.

This was his decision to be able to continue working in his profession while taking a medication that for almost everyone causes substantial weight gain. Even in the context of some medication-caused weight gain, changes in lifestyle can overcome at least a degree of it.

> •Insulin. Insulin is released automatically in your body after eating sugar or carbohydrates in order to lower blood sugar. It balances blood sugar and it also communicates that carbohydrates and sugar in your blood should be converted to fat for storage; thus, increased insulin levels will lead to increased fat storage. For individuals who have diabetes and are dependent on insulin, they will have to take this medication in order to remain alive, so if you are prescribed insulin, continue to take it but be aware that if the insulin levels are too high or if they are not properly managed, they may lead to increased weight gain.

> •Antipsychotic medications. These medications are tricky. They include such things as Zyprexa, Abilify, Seroquel, and a host of others. The challenge in identifying them is you may be prescribed an antipsychotic medication and not know that you are prescribed an antipsychotic medication. These medications are no longer just used to treat schizophrenia, they are used as an augmentation for depression treatment, they are

used to treat bipolar disorder, they may be used to treat some personality disorders, and other doctors may actually use them for sleep in low doses.

• Antidepressants are the next class of medication that tends to cause substantial weight gain, specifically those antidepressants that work on serotonin. Serotonin is one of the chemical systems in the brain that relates to aggression, anger, satiety, and depression, in addition to anxiety, so this group of antidepressants is often prescribed for anxiety as well as depression. Although many individuals will lose weight in the first six months while taking these medications, after the first six months, the weight tends to return and it usually returns in an amount far more than was lost in the first six months. Again, if you are being treated for a severe depression or other condition that requires this medication, do not abruptly stop it as these medications do have substantial side effects when abruptly discontinued, but do discuss with your physician whether an antidepressant with a different mechanism of action might be appropriate for you as serotonergic agents may make it more difficult to have successful weight loss.

• The next group of medications known to cause weight gain is mood stabilizers which includes Depakote, lithium, and most of the antiepileptic drugs which are also one of the other key groups that cause weight gain.

•Migraine medications also have the possibility of causing weight gain, especially those that are of the antidepressant class, such as tricyclic-type antidepressants.

•Another prominent medication that causes weight gain is any form of oral steroid medications, corticosteroids, such as prednisone. If your doctor prescribes a five-day Dosepak of Solu-Medrol to help you get over an infection, the five days of oral steroid is not going to cause substantial weight gain as it will be out of your body quite rapidly after the five-day course of treatment. However, long-term prescription of corticosteroid medication can cause substantial weight gain. Again, this may be medically necessary for conditions such as asthma or other conditions that require medications that reduce swelling; however, speak with your doctor about the possibility of another class of medication which will be less likely to cause weight gain as a side effect.

•Beta-blockers, which are used for blood pressure control and occasionally for the treatment of certain forms of anxiety, also are known to be substantial contributors to weight gain. Do not stop any medication designed to control your blood pressure without speaking to a primary care physician first as elevated blood pressure can become quite dangerous. There are other medications for blood pressure control which your physician may be able to recommend to you.

Finally, to end the top eight would be contraceptive medications which have a hormonal base within them.

Top Medical Conditions that Cause Weight Gain

If you have been diagnosed with one of these conditions, merely having the condition will put you at risk for substantial weight gain, and therefore it is important to get the condition treated appropriately by your medical doctor.

•The most common of these conditions is hypothyroidism. The thyroid is a gland located in your neck which releases thyroid hormones. These hormones go throughout the entire body and affect every cell. If your thyroid gland is sluggish and not putting out enough thyroid hormone, weight gain is an automatic result of this condition. If you are concerned about the possibility of having this condition, it will require a blood test from your physician in order to assess the functioning of your thyroid gland. Individuals with hypothyroidism will have an additional challenge in losing weight until their thyroid levels have normalized.

•Although it may be counterintuitive, the diagnosis of depression is associated with weight gain. There is a subgroup of people who are depressed who eat much less than average and will lose weight, but there is also a subgroup of individuals with depression who eat more than normal in order to make the depression feel better. Combined with eating more for comfort, they tend to exercise less because they have low energy levels. Depression should be evaluated either by a psychiatrist or family physician to see if treatment would be appropriate as it will be difficult to not only exercise but to complete the psychological experiences within this book if you are substantially depressed.

•Cushing's syndrome is a hormonal abnormality related to the excess of cortisol hormones in the body, and like individuals who have to take corticosteroids for a medical condition, the excess cortisol in the body causes substantial weight gain, usually in the face, neck, upper back, trunk, and abdomen; whereas, the hands and the legs remain thin. It is a unique pattern, and the risk of developing this syndrome is elevated in individuals with type 2 diabetes.

•Chronic stress can lead to weight gain.

•Polycystic ovary syndrome is another medical condition which leads to substantial weight gain.

Manage each and every one of these medical conditions or discuss the medications above with your physician in order to give you the best opportunity to successfully progress in your weight loss goals.

Physical Honesty

Remember, I noted earlier that we were going to engage in brutal self-honesty and exploration, and here is the beginning of the first part.

It is necessary, in order to obtain the information to move forward, that you know the amount of calories your body needs each and every day. In the past, the only way to accomplish this was to go into a medical facility, be submerged in a tank of water and have a series of biometric measures made which was intrusive, difficult, and not even available in many cities within the United States.

Today, there is a very simple way to accomplish this which I would recommend very highly, and that is purchasing either a FitBit or a BodyBugg. The FitBit simply fits in your pocket and monitors all of your movements throughout the day. The BodyBugg goes on a band around your arm and requires skin contact throughout the day. Both of them measure the number of calories that you exert in a day, and they upload it to their respective websites.

At the time that this book is being written, the website access is free for life for either of these products such that you can use it forever. The first time that you log into the website, you will put your name, age, weight, and height, and the computer will make an estimate of your daily caloric needs; however, as the days progress and you continue to enter weights over time, the program will adjust and actually demonstrate the calories that you actually burn each day at a particular weight. This is of inestimable value.

The most useless piece of information that doctors give on an hourly basis is "just cut back." If you do not know how much you have to cut back, you can never reach the goal of hitting the sweet spot in terms of calorie intake where you are getting enough to feel satisfied but not overshooting it to the mark of causing further weight gain, but also not going under the mark where you feel hungry all the time.

The second step of this process is keeping a food log, and this is very nicely tied in to your FitBit or BodyBugg in that when you go to your page at FitBit or BodyBugg, you have the opportunity to log your food for everything eaten during the day. It does neither you, nor anyone else, a service to leave things out because you do not want to divulge that giant chocolate cake that followed dinner.

The computer cannot assess your needs, and you cannot assess your needs, if it does not know about the cake, and you are the only one who has access to your page, so no one else has to know, but at least you have to know.

My recommendation is as you start into this, buy a small kitchen scale and weigh your food. I swear to you, if you look at a piece of steak, you cannot tell whether it is four ounces, six ounces or eight ounces by mere inspection. You must weigh it until you get a good visual sense, but if you are in a restaurant and you have a portion of food and you do not know exactly how much it was and you think maybe it is four ounces, maybe it is five ounces, when you log your food into the web site, put in six ounces.

Your goal in this process is to successfully lose weight, so if you are unsure, always estimate the food portion on the high side so that you do not undercount calories at the end of the day.

The other piece of information that supports my suggestion is that every study that has ever looked at our capacity to effectively evaluate the amount of food that we have eaten states that we always underestimate food portions when we guess about them later. Overcome this by knowing that that is a human blind spot, and *overestimate*.

If you have taken off your BodyBugg or your FitBit and you have engaged in some exercise, you can also add the exercise into the website and, therefore, get credit for it, but if you are going to estimate exercise, *underestimate* the number of miles you walked such that, again, at the end of the day, you will see a balance which will be promoting of weight loss.

The general goal with these plans is to eat 500 calories less than needed, and the program will automatically provide the number of calories by simply entering a goal into the program. The 500-per-day calorie deficit is automatically provided in the daily calorie allowance. A 500-calorie deficit each day of the week will result, on average, in a one-pound-per-week weight loss. The key word in that last sentence was "average."

Plan to enter food after breakfast and lunch, so that there will be clear indication of calories remaining at dinner, to stay within that calorie range rather than exceeding it. This is giving the strength of information, in the amount of food that will comply with the weight loss goal.

Exercise is important. I have noticed on those days when I sit in the office listening all day, compared to those days when I am walking between hospital wards and emergency rooms, I gain approximately 200 calories of activity when I am on the days walking versus the days sitting.

Exercise is not the entire piece of this picture because if I devoured a giant piece of chocolate cake that was 600 calories, it would take an inordinate amount of exercise to burn those 600 calories within the day. Just because we are getting a few extra calories by walking a little bit more, that does not open the door to giant intake of wildly inappropriate foods.

EXPERIENCE #2: GO TO YOUR LOCAL BOOKSTORE AND BROWSE THE DIET SECTION

Pick up books from all of the major diet systems - Weight Watchers, low-fat diets, low-carb diets, The Mediterranean Diet, The Atkins Diet – and peruse the book section where the meal plans are located. Read a week's worth of the suggested meals for that diet. Make a list of those foods on a paper that you take with you or on a page in the Action Book.

Sit down afterwards and do a deeply honest appraisal

with yourself. Chose which one of these meal plans you could envision living with, with some degree of modification at a later point, but in general the type of meal plan that you could envision eating starting today and continuing for years.

My wife is a delightful person who could not eat a diet that did not include fresh fruit no matter what its benefits were. If someone were to suggest to her any other form of diet, it would be ignored before the first meal of the plan was warm.

I am an individual who prefers to eat meats and cheeses, and so a diet which eliminated those things entirely would not be on the table for me irrespective of any other issues. For me, a low-carbohydrate diet has been highly successful. For my wife, a low-fat diet is highly successful.

There is no right diet for everyone, but there is a diet that you will be able to tolerate as opposed to a diet that you will not be able to tolerate, and your job in this experience is to find the diet that will most closely fit your basic food loves. If you find the diet while you are still sitting in the bookstore, then go ahead and grab that book because that is the one that you will be using for your actual diet plan.

Psychological Honesty

Now we approach the real core of this book. Everything has been in preparation to this point, which was necessary. We are, in psychiatric terms, biological, psychological, social, and spiritual beings, and the first portion of this book has been looking a lot at the biological part of diet, the biological part of who you are, and ways that you can keep your biological self as healthy as possible so that the other parts of you can be happy and joyful as a result and can live as long as possible.

This book is not going to talk any more about what diet you should follow, how many hours a day you should exercise. That is finished.

We are going to examine the history of your eating behavior as it is a lifelong pattern, since it is, and we are going to use a metaphor of a long, energetic string which is of a particular shape. The length of this string goes back through your entire life. The shape of the string is particular to you and was molded by life experience. It attracts certain experiences to it, and rejects others. We will simply call these experiences pearls, and these particular pearls have a hollowed-out section that matches the shape of your string.

As you have eating experiences, whether it is delight at eating your favorite dessert or the shame of stepping on a scale, they all have some aspect that fits on this lifelong pattern encoded into the dynamic string.

Many people have successfully lost weight in the past using any kind of diet, and they fit into that perfect outfit to go to the prom, to go to the children's graduation or the class reunion to look perfect and two weeks later rebound back to a weight that was higher than they had ever imagined their weight could have gone. The reason is they exerted a degree of willpower to successfully lose weight for a specific purpose, but they did not identify the string, they did not remove any pearls – they simply started putting new pearls back on the string of bad eating behavior as soon as the special event ended.

This book is going to aid you in transforming the shape and energy of the string thereby removing the old pearls and creating entirely new ones more in line with your conscious plans.

EXPERIENCE #3: THE WEIGH-IN

I want you to take a day in which you do not have a lot of other pressing engagements. Take an area of the house that will be private and weigh yourself at least every two hours while you are awake. Weigh before you eat, after you eat, naked, clothed, shoes on, shoes off – it does not matter. Simply get as many weights onto this page as you can fit.

Take the highest weight on that page, subtract the lowest weight on the page, and that is your weight variance.

If you have a weight change that is within this weight variance, then you can make some adjustments in your assessment of success. For example, if you have to weigh wearing your clothes one day, you will have a sense of how much your clothes weigh so that if you are up a pound wearing your clothes, you will know that was your clothes. It was not that you gained weight or that you failed on your diet.

You need to have a sense of this variance because our weight will change by several pounds throughout the day.

Weight Schedule during Weight Loss

Based upon the experience just finished, one of the key pieces to learn from this is that you should weigh at the same time every day to the degree possible in order to cut out the variance you may see at different points during the day.

The second thing you should do is plan to weigh naked so that you do not have the variation of different clothes at different times of the year or different shoes at different times of the year. You are attempting to weigh you, not the accoutrements that you wear in your daily life.

Next, follow the diet plan that you have chosen, follow the plan exactly, and we will deal with issues that come up if there are challenges later in the book. After you have made your initial weight, plan to weigh every few weeks as you continue through the diet plan.

This sounds counterintuitive; however, if you truly have a 500-calorie deficit each day and you follow the plan of your diet, whether it be low-fat or low-carbohydrate, you will in fact lose weight. It is a physiological requirement. However, the weight on the scale may, oddly enough, not change and that is because of other factors.

You may be changing some of your fat cells and building muscle cells. Muscle weighs more than fat, unit per unit; thus, you may actually appear to have gained weight by stepping on the scale, whereas in fact you have lost several pounds of body fat and are more healthy; thus, do not weigh too often as long as you are willing to follow the diet plan. That way, you are sure to see success when you weigh at a later point in time. Sometimes the scale seems "stuck" for several weeks during a weight plateau, but will then drop several pounds seemingly all at once.

My recommendation for frequency of weights will change markedly when we move into the maintenance phase after successful weight loss.

Consider purchasing a scale that measures body fat, or BMI, in addition to total weight. The reason for this is if you see a decrease in your BMI, this is a success, much as finding your clothes are fitting more loosely, a major success which may not immediately be reflected in the number of weight itself.

If you break your diet for some reason, make that diet break a one-meal break only. Do not tell yourself that because you ate this nice dessert at lunch, you might as well have something else at dinner. Rather, acknowledge that you had the food at lunch but that you are going to return to your diet at dinner so that the one error does not create a substantial compounding of problems. And do not forget to forgive and love yourself. We all make mistakes on any diet occasionally, and that is OK when they remain single mistakes.

Chapter Four

Universal Fantasy

Not *That* Kind of Fantasy

When psychiatrists use the term "fantasy," we are typically referring to an internal type of belief that is fixed and unchanging when it has not been clearly examined or brought to the light of conscious awareness. This is different from simply a belief system which may also resist change until brought to light because the fantasy structure usually has some area of unreality attached to it.

Forever Thin

The universal fantasy all of us who have failed at diets share is: "When I finish my diet, I will eat anything I want again, and I will stay at my goal weight." Some people might actually define this in the colloquial sense of insanity; that is, expecting different results to occur from the same actions that failed in the past.

The key problem with this internal fantasy is that it leads to a pattern called "yo-yo dieting," in which people successfully lose weight when they have a high motivation to do so and then after coming off the diet will be so relieved that they eat any- and everything, leading not only the weight that they lost to come back, but also additional weight as well.

One of the biological imperatives that follows from the notion of the body being designed to store fat is that in situations where we lose weight, our body's initial signal is to attempt to get the weight back, especially to store the fat back, and so once eating returns, the body will become more efficient and it will store more fat, even from almost the same calorie load as previously.

Without commitment or interest in a long-term solution, it is best not to engage in short-term dieting followed by yo-yos, as this only causes additional problems.

Consciousness Cures

Ken Wilbur, a notable writer in the area of consciousness and meditation, stated that when people become fully conscious of anything, it ceases to become a major problem. Many people who are struggling with weight will respond with, "I know I am fat. What are you talking about? I am conscious of being fat – just look at me!"

This is not what I mean by the term "consciousness." You may be aware that you are overweight, people may tell you that, you may see it in the mirror, but that is not the same thing as becoming fully conscious of the problem.

The degree of reaching consciousness about weight or any other major life problem is to fully experience both the overweightness and all of the causes, issues, problems, emotions, and life stories that led to the overweightness, and as the light shines through the darkness and illuminates those cobwebs, they will cease to affect you in the way that they have up until the present.

The goal is to identify patterns of feelings and understandings, and that is what we will be doing when we reach Chapter Seven. Resistance equals repetition.

One of the most profound psychiatrists I can identify, Dr. Carl Jung, noted that the goal of personal growth is to bring material that was unconscious into consciousness, and the failure to do so will cause the person to view problems in life as the result of fate external to themselves.

In this course of brutal self-honesty, our goal is to find the psychological truths that lead to the behavior that we want to change. Fighting the awareness of these truths causes them to become more resistant, just like the yo-yo diet, because they get buried a little bit more deeply, and these unconscious pieces of material will cause repetition of the unhealthy behavior.

As Dr. Jung pointed out, often rather than taking responsibility for these blind spots (these areas that we are unaware of), we instead view them as fate or something that was controlled by outside of ourselves – things like, "I would have stayed on my diet had my wife not brought home my favorite pie. How could I possibly have resisted that?"

This kind of statement relinquishes power to the other person or event rather than claiming it for yourself. Claiming your power, though, entails the responsibility of considering whether you might potentially survive skipping the pie.

EXPERIENCE #4: PHYSICAL BLINDSPOTS

In medical school, we learned that each eye has a physiological blind spot, and we each experienced it, yet this exercise has wowed rooms of physicians.

Take the first figure that is attached here. You will see a dot and a cross. Close your left eye and focus on the cross on the paper in front of you with your right eye. Move it forward and backward until the dot completely disappears. At a particular length from your face, probably somewhere between six and fourteen inches, you will not see the dot even though it is on the paper.

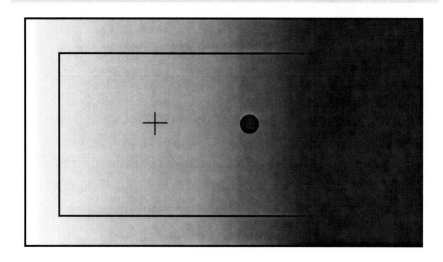

This is an example and a description of the physiological blind spot at the back of your eye where the optic nerve leaves; however, that is not the magic of what you are experiencing. The magic of what you are experiencing is the fact that your conscious awareness and brain are actually filling in that black spot with what they believe should be there, which is the area surrounding it. You are getting a false interior experience of the image because in fact a black spot exists in that location, but your eye cannot see it.

Likewise, look at the additional diagrams and download free ones from www.newmindnewbody.com that are in color, and you will be able to observe not only does your consciousness fill in the spot, it will also fill in gradients, colors, patterns, images, and even gross representations of text in an attempt to fill this space that it cannot see.

In real life, your brain fills in the blind spot every instant, but it does have help. The two things that help your brain do that more effectively is the fact that you have another eye, presumably, and it is looking at the same information from a different angle, thereby providing data for brain to process.

The second way that we deal with this physiological blind spot is to move our eyes nearly constantly. It is exceptionally rare that we focus on any one object and not move our eyes for an extended period; thus, the microscopic eye movements going back and forth will help fill in those pieces of the blind spot, again providing the extra data to the brain.

This is an important model to consider because we are going to be using this very same experiential metaphor to look at your psychological blind spots by looking at them from different vantage points, different angles, and hopefully as moving targets.

Psychological Blind Spots

All of us who have had problems or difficulties with weight have psychological blind spots surrounding weight which we ignore because we do not know what they are.

The exercises that follow are designed to start illuminating these blind spots so that you can bring the light of consciousness to transform them with the experiences described later in the book. This is the process of revealing the metaphorical string and the metaphorical pearls that I have been describing.

Chapter Five

The Hypnotic Mind

Models are Models

Alfred Korzybski, the father of general semantics, famously said, "The map is not the territory." The profundity of his statement is beyond the scope of this discussion, but the key is to realize that reality is larger than any single model invoked to explain it. There are many models of the mind; however, none of them contain all of the explanatory information about the mind. The topic is too complex for any single model to encompass.

You can consider this very much like a map you might purchase. If you wanted to hike in the mountains, you would want a map of hiking trails. In order to follow the trail to your destination, a weather map might be useful to you, but it would not show you where to walk. Likewise, a tourist map of a destination might give you interesting places to visit as a tourist, but it would not necessarily help you find real estate. We have to choose our maps carefully and use the ones that will help us get to our destination.

Psychology and psychiatry have multiple different maps of the mind. One of the most common ones currently is a cognitive behavioral model which examines cognitive schema to explain various psychological phenomena. However, this is not the model that will be most useful for us as we begin to explore eating behavior and changing unconscious wishes. It is not wrong it just does not address the areas of the mind we need to explore.

We will be looking at the hypnotic mind as a particular model which will allow for change in lifelong patterns. This chapter will describe the model of the hypnotic mind and a little bit about how it functions, which we will use in later chapters.

Hypnosis and psychiatry have had a very interesting and intertwined history over the course of centuries. I will not belabor the entire event; however, I would point out that a young, budding neurologist named Dr. Sigmund Freud traveled to Paris to work with the leading neurologist of his time, Dr. Eugene Marie Charcot.

Charcot was finding a series of patients who had anesthesia and paralysis in various parts of their bodies that the new science of neurology could not begin to understand because the symptoms did not match the pattern of nerve distribution to the regions of the body. Charcot and others began to name this phenomenon "hysteria." The current term for this condition is "conversion disorder" in the American system of psychiatric diagnosis.

This amazing clinical entity, which is still observable today, became a focus of Sigmund Freud's work. Charcot and others were using hypnosis to treat this condition with great effect other than some difficulties with symptom substitution in some cases. Freud became uncomfortable with hypnosis and developed psychoanalysis as an alternative means of accessing the unconscious.

Charcot was one of the leading proponents of hypnosis of his day. He oddly enough ended up being entirely wrong in nearly all of his assumptions about hypnosis as a state of consciousness, however. His compatriot, Dr. Hippolyte Bernheim, at the Nancie Institute in France, actually formed a far more coherent version of hypnosis, far more congruent with our understanding today.

Two primary theorists in the mid-twentieth century of hypnosis are the people whose ideas we will most closely follow. One was Dave Elman, who worked in stage hypnosis as a young man and developed rapid induction techniques.

Rapid access to a trance state is essential for us because the induction techniques used at the time of Freud and Bernheim could take as long as two hours to hypnotize a patient. We need to accomplish this in a matter of minutes; otherwise, it would not be time efficient for any of us. David Elman brought this method of rapid induction into use, and he taught physicians for decades in his method.

There exist DVDs and videos in which Dave Elman and his students used his induction to promote surgical anesthesia for patients who did not require any other form for chemical anesthesia for major surgical operations. This demonstrates the depth of the power of hypnotic trance when the state reached is a deep enough one to make profound personal change.

The other notable hypnotist in the twentieth century was psychiatrist Dr. Milton Erickson. He used a nonformal trance induction method as he assumed people were in a trance all the time anyway, and he would make nondirective permissive kinds of interventions. This is much more difficult to teach; however, there will be a few experiences in this and later chapters which will allow you to use some of his ideas effectively as well. In addition, the neurolinguistic programming techniques which are later in this book are based upon the Ericksonian principles of hypnosis.

Model of the Hypnotic Mind

In the traditional sense, the mind is broken into three categories in the hypnotic model. The first is the conscious mind, the second is the unconscious mind, and the third is what I call the physical monitoring area. As a caveat, many hypnotists use the term "subconscious" rather than "unconscious," but as a psychiatrist, I am more comfortable with the latter phrase. Feel free to substitute the terms.

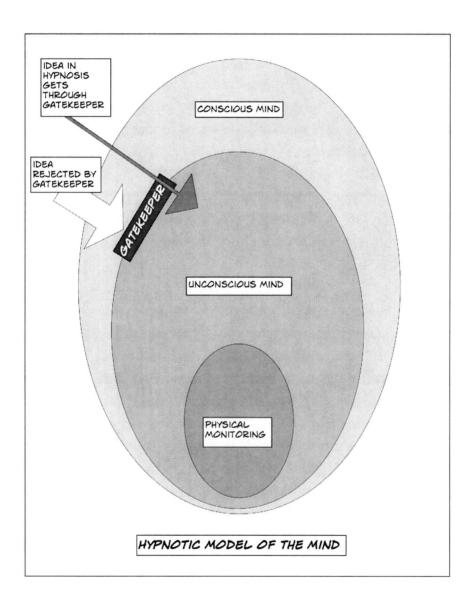

The conscious mind is the level of our experience that includes logic, willpower, surface interactions with others, rational choice, and short-term memory.

The unconscious mind contains longstanding patterns of emotional and behavioral patterns that evolve over time. It is automatic, and generally resistant to change. Long-term memory resides here.

The physical monitoring layers of the mind are those areas which relate to maintaining blood pressure, immune function and other automatic functions that we typically have little awareness over.

The key factor in change, according to this hypnotic model, is changing the longstanding patterns and assumptions that exist in the unconscious mind. This is not as easily accomplished as only repeating a simple affirmation, although there is nothing wrong with repeating affirmations.

The reason for this is that many of the patterns in our unconscious mind may have been heard or internally repeated many hundreds of thousands of repetitions over the course of a lifetime. For example: "I feel fat." "I am not attractive enough." "What is wrong with me?" "Why do people not find me attractive?"

The automatic underlying thoughts and the emotions that go with them have so many repetitions to back them up that stating an affirmation such as, "I am beautiful and healthy," is generally ignored at the deeper layers of the mind. Although it does make the conscious mind very happy, it does not necessarily cause any internal change.

There is a gatekeeper, or sensor, which actually prevents this material from reaching the unconscious. By having such low abilities in regular life to get these new fresh ideas into the unconscious, change becomes more difficult.

Hypnosis is a particular state of mind in which the body is relaxed but the mind is focused in a manner that allows you to bypass the gatekeeper. Once you can bypass the gatekeeper, you can implant new things in and you can get old stuff out of the unconscious.

That is the special and unique focus of the hypnotic mind that is not necessarily present in regular meditative states, or relaxed states, certainly not present when you are working away at a job or attempting to do things at a highly conscious level.

Rules of the Hypnotic Mind

Every thought or idea causes some physical reaction. Although this is most dramatic in the cases of hypnotic-induced anesthesia for surgery, as an example given earlier, this also occurs on more subtle levels in which a thought or idea accepted by the unconscious mind will lead to differences in physical reactions, for example, to food or other experiences.

It is easy to demonstrate in hypnotic states, for example,

an allergic reaction to a drop of water and then remove it just as easily through suggestion alone. These are physical reactions that happen immediately and directly when in this particular state of mind.

Once an idea is accepted by the unconscious mind, it remains until replaced by something else. As I noted earlier, the unconscious mind is very much automatic and tends to resist change. That is why patterns that started early in childhood may persist into adulthood if they are not examined and brought to the light of consciousness.

Once they are changed and accepted by the unconscious mind, the new material will stay there until it is itself changed, meaning that once you have fixed a particular pattern or problem, it will stay fixed and you do not have to continue to revisit it indefinitely.

Each suggestion acted upon creates less opposition. This is used in the course of the induction that we will practice later. For example, when recommendations that you become more relaxed or more peaceful are acted upon, then later suggestions regarding weight or other activities will be more readily accepted, mostly because you accepted the first.

Key point: When we do the induction later, play along with it. If you fight each one of the words in the induction, then you will fight the suggestions that you want to give to yourself later. If you play along and have fun with it, your unconscious mind is much more likely to accept the suggestions when they occur.

In dealing with the unconscious, the greater amount of conscious effort there is, the less the unconscious response. This is exemplified by the yo-yo diet and the problems that go with it. We put every ounce of conscious effort into losing weight and then it immediately bounces back thereafter the minute we let our conscious awareness slip away from that focus.

If, instead of putting all of that effort into the diet and putting more effort into unconscious change, then the diet becomes an automatic response to the new person whom you have become.

Imagination is more powerful than knowledge when dealing with the unconscious. When you go to buy a car, the salesman, if they are well trained, does not sit and give you a series of informational points about a car, such as, this is how much it weighs, this is how fast it goes, this is how much the fuel tank holds. Instead, they begin to engage your imagination by saying things like, "Can you imagine driving this car down the road and how you might feel, what it would be like to put the top down on the convertible?"

As they engage the imagination, it is changing your unconscious in terms of your initial plan of buying a car that day in a way that the dry statistics of the vehicle would have failed to do.

EXPERIENCE #5: WILLPOWER LOST

Take a moment and document the last diet that you were on. Document what you did, how much weight you lost, how long it took you, what it was like and ultimately document the event that led you to leave the diet. The event that led to leaving the diet can almost always be characterized as a failure of willpower.

Why Willpower Always Loses

Willpower is an awesome part of our being and it has the capacity in the short term to prevent falling off the diet path. However, relying on willpower for long-term change will always fail, and the reason this is true is elucidated in the hypnotic mind model.

Willpower is an aspect of the conscious mind. It requires considerable effort, control, and it also tends to weaken when we have additional external stress, things going on that are bothering us, work going badly, relationships going badly – willpower for diet will become weaker at that point.

The lifelong patterns that have developed in the unconscious mind, however, have much more strength and they also have the staying power of a lifetime; thus, they will eventually win in the battle of will versus desire. Changing the patterns in the unconscious and removing those negative aspects is the only way to create long-term change.

Chuck exemplifies the strength of the unconscious winning over willpower. He had already had surgery to remove his entire stomach several years prior. After the surgery he successfully lost over 150 pounds, and was pleased with his success. He experienced feelings of deprivation eating the microscopic portions required after this surgery. He discovered that if he ate a bit more at each meal, he could hold down that extra food without feeling nausea. Over time, he had stretched his intestines back into a pouch that resembled a stomach enough that he could eat larger portions of food. He gained all the weight lost, even without a stomach! Even a total gastrectomy could not overcome his lifelong patterns of eating behavior.

BEHAVIOR TIP #2: EAT YOUR LAST MEAL OF THE DAY BEFORE 6:00 P.M. AND EAT NOTHING THEREAFTER

Your body is designed to retain and promote fat retention, and after eating a meal, you will have additional calories. If you eat too late in the evening and then go to sleep soon thereafter, your body has no choice but to turn all of those additional calories into fat because there has been nothing that has occurred to burn the calories.

This is true even if you have had a high-protein snack in the evening because protein can be converted to sugar through gluconeogenesis, and any sugar eaten in the evening will automatically turn to fat unless there has been exercise after the sugar intake that will burn those calories.

Eating your final meal earlier in the evening allows

more time for activity to occur and thereby reduce the amount of food that might be transformed into fat.

EXPERIENCE #6: HYPNOTIC MIND RECALL

This is fun, and it illustrates what I have been discussing about the hypnotic mind and how certain information comes so readily in the form of impulse and pattern and not so much in the form of knowledge.

Take a moment and think to some time in your childhood when you heard a jingle from a commercial that will instantly come back into your mind. The one that comes to my mind is the Tic-Tac commercial from the mid-1970s: "Put a Tic-Tac in your mouth and get a bang out of life." This comes instantly without thought. It goes through every level of the gatekeeper with no problem. It got into deep layers of mind, and it comes out equally as easy. Write it down quickly.

From the same time period that you remember the jingle from your childhood, as quickly write down who the vice president of the United States was. More of a challenge? The reason this is more difficult is the vice president requires accessing knowledge. The jingle came automatically because it was specifically designed to affect you at an unconscious level, and this is the power of the hypnotic model of the mind. Marketers use these techniques with great success. After all, if you are humming the "Tic-Tac" song, or it is popping into your mind, what are you likely to buy the next time you are in the grocery store?

Chapter Six

Overdetermined Behavior

What Is It?

The previously mentioned Dr. Sigmund Freud eventually became a psychiatrist and the developer of psychoanalysis rather than becoming the neurologist that he had originally planned. Although not all of the ideas and notions that Freud discussed were accurate, he was nevertheless a keen observer of human behavior and consciousness. He developed a series of methods of discovering patterns from the unconscious.

One of the key important points that came to me in the course of my own battles with impulses to eat and long-term weight control came from a frustration. This frustration was that I would try a series of psychological techniques that I had unearthed or found somewhere, and it would seem as if there was a shift in my perception towards food or towards weight.

Then I would notice that nothing had changed on the scales and nothing had really changed with regard to what I was choosing to eat even though something *felt* a little bit different. I contemplated what in the world could be leading to this after going through so much work and still finding failure at the end of it.

The "aha" moment came when the concept of overde-termination popped into my mind, which was one of the words that I learned back in my psychiatric residency.

Overdetermined behavior is almost like a condensation or a drop or a compromise between a whole host of different competing interests in the mind at the unconscious level, and this overdetermined behavior is like the perfect solution to all of these problems all at once.

The challenge is that the overdetermined behavior may not be a behavior that you want to use long term, but at the point it was created, it stuck, because it was so efficient. This is very different, for example, from the type of causation that we tend to talk about in the more modern world.

Let us take an example. If we observe four or five roads converging onto one another creating a traffic jam at the end of the road, we could reasonably hypothesize that if we blocked some of the feeder roads that the traffic jam would get better on the main road because we have reduced the amount of traffic flowing through. This would be a model of simple causation.

We might also see this in context of work environments where assessments are done to see how efficiency could be im-proved. They may suggest that if one part of the shipping pro-cess was improved, for example, there would be a ten percent improvement in timeliness.

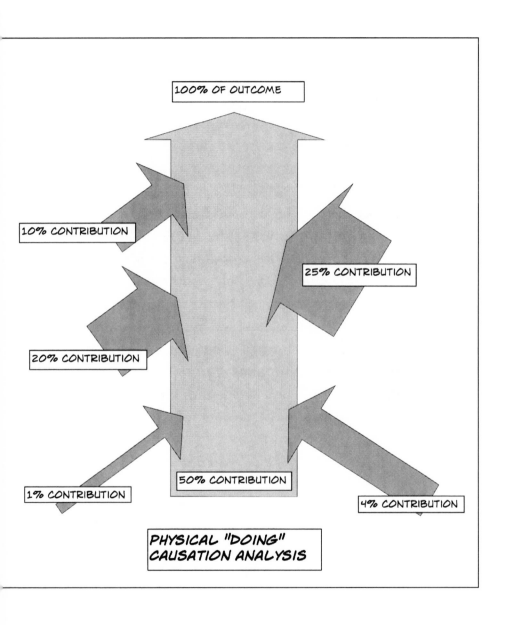

This is exactly what does *not* happen in overdetermined symptoms. These reside in a psychological reality which is based in the unconscious, not something conscious and measurable like the traffic example or the work efficiency example. An overdetermined behavior is fixing so many small things with one symptom that when you remove one of those small things, it does not affect the final symptom at all. In order to affect the eating behavior (which is the symptom), which is overdetermined, we must clear or transform a substantial number of the contributing factors rather than just a few of them.

The other interesting factor in overdetermination is we do not get a percent improvement by fixing small things. We experience the full problem until enough of the small pieces are altered to make the overdetermined symptom disappear and vanish. At the level of the association cortex in the brain, this is the step where the neuronal net rewires new meaning which separates eating from the reward system, discussed earlier.

Overdetermined symptoms are not just eating behavior and weight; they include any problem of life which feels particularly stuck in spite of multiple attempts to resolve or overcome.

EXPERIENCE #7: PAST ATTEMPTS

Describe in detail, not necessarily the most recent, but the most significant of your past attempts at long-term weight loss. Describe the feelings that you experienced when you were successful at initially losing the weight. Then describe what feeling states started to arise after a bit of time occurred.

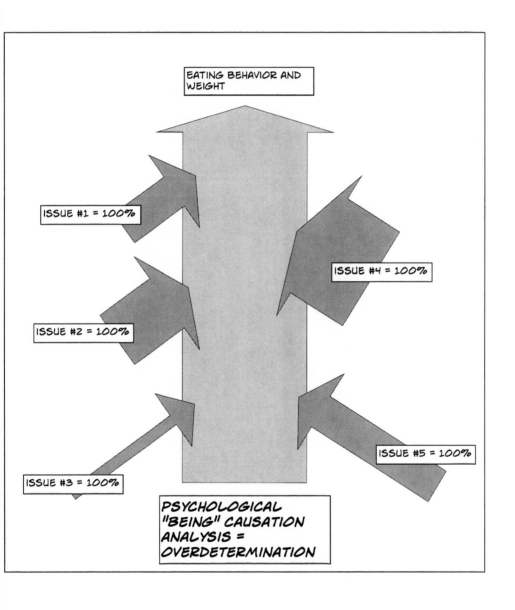

Using this as a template, describe several other of your attempts and the feeling states during, right after, and then a bit after your weight loss.

Can you discover any particular feeling states or anxieties that led you to return to unhealthy eating in the period after your successful weight loss? Write those feelings down; we will be using them in upcoming chapters.

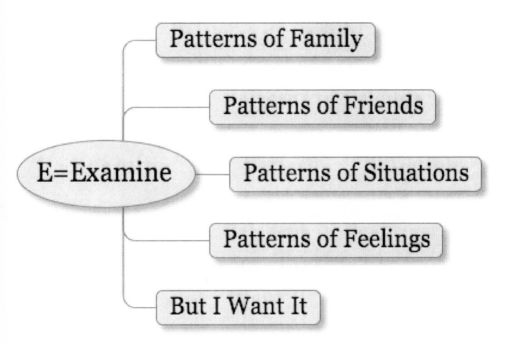

Chapter Seven

Mind Maps

In the 1970s, the Boeing 747 was the most complicated passenger aircraft built. The manuals designed to help the engineers learn the systems within the 747 spanned multiple volumes and took many months for engineers to master. Boeing underwent an experiment in which they used a mind map which circled the entire classroom and illustrated each of the major hydraulic and electrical systems in the 747 on this single very long page, and it reduced the learning time for the engineers from months to weeks.

Southwest Medical School has a counseling program in place for students. Medical students rarely have had the experience of failing anything in their lives because they had to succeed to a substantial degree to even get accepted into medical school, but it is in medical school that often those first difficulties occur in the basic science years. The counseling program for remediation of grades used mind mapping as the primary study tool for students who then often went from marginal grades to some of the best grades in the class, and there are several reasons for this.

Mind mapping is both a visual and a verbal medium in that it is using visuospatial information in the terms of the diagram, in which placement of items in their relationship to each other provides the visual gestalt. This is combined with short words or phrases that will help trigger complex ideas from just a small nugget of words.

This activates and allows for integration between verbal and nonverbal, left brain and right brain, parts and wholes, and the logical and the synthetic portions of the brain, all with one mapping modality. This unique property gives the mind map considerably more power in terms of understanding than, for example, an extended outline which could be another means of creating the same information set.

We can use mind maps to explore parts of ourselves and brainstorm information about ourselves and our life patterns. We can use anything in a mind map to illustrate the points being described, including photographs, diagrams, pictures, symbols, and words. The hallmark is to assemble it together into a whole so that we can see it as a whole in addition to the pieces.

The scribbled little diagram on a napkin at the dinner table is probably some variant of a mind map. This is an example of the low-tech version that you can use throughout the balance of this course whenever we talk about doing mind maps. There are also sophisticated, easy-to-navigate computer programs that generate mind maps you can change, update, and alter without having to start over on ink and paper.

EXPERIENCE #8: MIND MAP YOUR MOTHER

We will start with a mind-mapping exercise making your mother the central core of the mind map. Since this is just an exercise in looking at how to create a mind map and how to interlink the pieces together, Mom is usually a complicated enough topic for anyone to allow for some variety and some interesting things to emerge, part of which may relate to eating behavior since mothers and caring often relate to such.

Use the template that I have provided in the book. You can enlarge it or you can find the one in the Action Book, which will be a larger size, or make one of your own by hand. Make a line at the end of each final word in the chain and write anything that comes to your mind from your life experiences. Your added branches may fill the page!

Key things to note are the interrelationships between paths and how the paths interrelate to each other. We will begin using specific mind maps quite soon to illustrate each of the major areas where eating behavior may become problematic. We will then use the information from the mind map to engage in exercises to transform you.

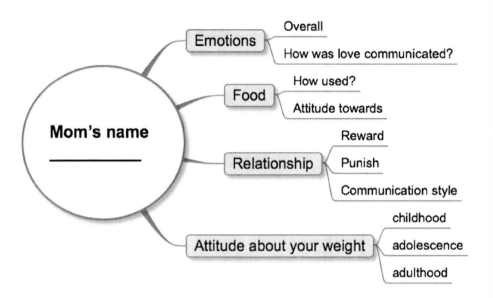

BEHAVIOR TIP #3: AFTER THE LAST MEAL OF THE DAY, ENGAGE IN SOME LIGHT EXERCISE TO BURN ABOUT 100 CALORIES

You do not want to engage in heavy exercise right before attempting to go to sleep as it may activate you so much that you cannot go to sleep; however, a short walk of 100 calories in the early evening will burn off excess carbohydrates, thereby preventing them being transformed into fat while you sleep.

It gives you a little bit of cushion at the end of the day if you are right at the edge in terms of your food diary calorie components and allows you to have a little bit more control over perhaps an appropriate treat at the end of dinner if you are willing to engage in that activity.

It also will help significantly with energy slumps that happen in the midevening because getting a few calories burned will give you additional energy and help you stay awake until the time you are ready to actually go to sleep for the evening.

Chapter Eight

Blame or No Blame?

It Is Really All about You

Blame is a deeply toxic emotion that erodes away the possibility of psychospiritual growth in life. Ultimately, it is up to each of us to decide whether to forgive others for their either real or imagined transgressions for the purpose of growing into a new person.

One of the primary difficulties with individuals stuck in a blame pattern is that they tend to believe that if they let go of the blame, it equates in some way to supporting the wrongdoing that someone else did to them and thereby promoting the behavior, when it was in fact a negative and hurtful behavior.

The truth, however, is that blame affects only one person in the world, and that is the one who holds it – you. The person whom you blame for something that happened in the past probably does not know you blame them, and if they do know, they likely do not care.

The blame that holds in anger, depression, hopelessness, and helplessness, all bundled together in a single sort of emotional state, is hurting you, potentially making you sick but certainly making you miserable. Letting go of it is something that can only be of help to you. Keeping it bound tight leads to increased feelings of powerlessness which, again, affects you, not the person who did the wrongdoing.

Example: Grandma's Love

Here is an innocuous example of this particular situation and the choices about blame that should be easy to follow and yet illustrate the core point that I am trying to make. The triviality of the example removes the emotional tone, without losing the idea.

My grandmother was the most wonderful person in my world as a child and I loved her dearly. She loved to cook as a way of expressing her love. She would make such things as sugar toast which was white bread with dollops of butter in each corner covered in white granular sugar and toasted. Obviously, potentially the worst food that could never fit on any diet at all, but perfectly delightful for a child to experience from his grandmother's kitchen.

She also had an incredible ability to make Crisco crusts that would be just so flaky they would melt in your mouth. She made a chicken pie with this crust that anyone would die for just to eat. I have never met anyone who could equal her in piecrust skills, and it has been many years.

Grandmothers and grandfathers always have the extraordinary luxury of handing children back to their parents after spoiling them, and of course grandma's overall love and caring was also transmitted through food, so one of the things that I learned, of course, was that food was a way to experience and share love from my grandmother.

My mother, of course, had the responsibility of making sure that the kids were healthy as opposed to just delighted with what they were eating, and so she would insist that we eat things like celery. But comparing celery to sugar toast; that is not even in the same ballpark of choices for a kid.

It is an interesting dynamic, and looking back upon it, I could, of course, in some way try to blame my grandmother for feeding me too much sugar at various points in life. But I would not choose to because she was acting out of love and caring. If I chose to blame her for growing up with a "sweet tooth" I would actually only be hurting myself because I would have given away all of my personal power and responsibility over my current food choices. The simple fact is that at the point I understood anything about food, it became my responsibility to choose properly, not the fault of anyone else.

In certain family situations, things that happen in the past may feel as if they deserve more blame, but nevertheless, as we become adults and look back upon these particular circumstances, we have the capacity to let go of blame and yet retain the feelings that are associated, and with my grandmother, those feelings have always been loving and positive.

Observing Yourself as if from Afar

One of the challenges in order to let go of blame and to let go of other emotions is the capacity to begin observing yourself as if you were a third person.

This is actually the core of several different meditative practices that are cultivated in different traditions, specifically called "mindfulness"; however, without going that far into the notion, simply taking a step back rather than reacting to a situation is a great start. If we can hold onto the thought or the feeling and observe it for a period of time, identify it and write it down, we have stopped the chain reaction of simple, mindless responses to feelings.

There will be a meditative practice in one of the next chapters called "Thoughts as Bubbles," which will help you begin to develop this practice quite easily and give you a sense of what it is like to examine stressful situations, or any other situations, without fully identifying with them.

Once we have the capacity to observe things from this third-person perspective, it is easier to begin to let go of the kinds of emotions that gnaw away at our core, such as blame. It is essential not to attempt to push all of your feelings aside; however, it is possible to feel the negative consequences of a past act or a past unpleasant experience without necessarily involving blame because the blame, as I noted above, makes us powerless in the situation and traps us in yet more negative feelings.

Chapter Nine

Patterns of Family

Some of our earliest experiences in life related to eating and food and the feelings that we mix with them come from early family experiences. Some dinner tables are pleasant places where people discuss the events of the day and create a very positive sense towards food. Other dinner tables define open warfare and connect food with very negative feelings.

This creates a very complicated patchwork quilt that develops over the course of time in how eating behavior evolves. The purpose of this chapter and the purpose of the task here is to begin to identify each of those threads, each of the pieces of the patchwork, so that we can begin to examine what defined your internal string which holds the pearls. This is where you start with the real challenges of the hero's journey.

We are going to complete a mind map for each of the family members with whom you grew up. It is important to note that you may have an evolving set of feelings over the course of childhood and adolescence, in which case you can note at what age the feeling state began to change and what the relationship was with food when it did change.

EXPERIENCE #9: MIND MAP THE FAMILY

Allow yourself a moment of silence and quietly ask yourself who the most important person in your past was who influenced your eating patterns and your concept of weight and self. Allow the first impression to enter your awareness and write down their name and their relation to you in the center of the mind map.

Now fill out the questions and anything that comes to mind for each of the branches on the mind map pattern that is present on this page. To make this a bit easier, simply write over any of the branches which are only labeled "topic." You can add more branches, but at least three for each subheading such as "incidents of note."

After you complete this exercise with the first family member, repeat the exercise until you have completed a mind map for each of the people who were primary in your family of origin, the family that you grew up with in your home. If an uncle came for Thanksgiving and said something hateful to you that stuck with you the rest of your life, include one for him as well because that is a notable experience that goes beyond the nuclear family but something which is a stain in your consciousness.

Continue doing mind maps on each of the family members and family groups until you have exhausted anything that comes to mind in terms of food, eating, and family relationships.

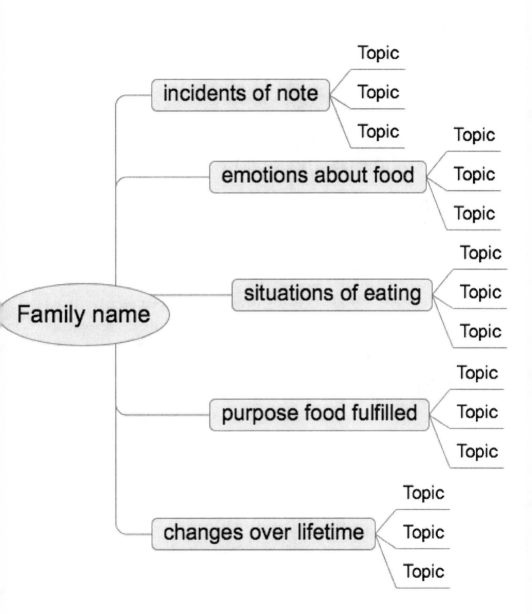

At the end of this exercise, review all of the mind maps you have created and look over them to see if there is a particular emotional pattern or an age pattern that comes to mind that has led to your behaviors related to eating or to weight. Make a list of those on a separate piece of paper, and we will utilize them in a later chapter.

BEHAVIOR TIP #4: WHEN YOU HAVE THE OPPORTUNITY, TAKE THE STAIRS

If you have not climbed stairs in years, then do not climb to the seventeenth floor the first time you try this. Use common sense and start with the number of stairs that are comfortable for you to accomplish. At work or in hotels or if on vacation, take the stairs instead of using the elevators. People pay money to use Stairmasters in the gym, when stairs exist all over the place that can be used for free.

These exercises and increases in physical activity throughout the day can give you several hundred extra calories burned if done on a consistent basis. Another simple task: when you park your car, park in the middle of the parking lot rather than at the space closest to the door. Those few extra steps help.

You can monitor this with your BodyBugg or your Fit-Bit, and you will notice a change in caloric use if you engage in some of these minor activities spread throughout the day.

The other benefit of increasing your activity to a degree

in the middle of the day is you will begin to increase your base metabolism rate so that you will burn a few extra calories even when you are not exercising.

Chapter Ten

Patterns of Friends

L ike the previous chapter, we will examine the relationships with people who have been close to you throughout your life. Family patterns tend to be highly instructive for early ages up until about adolescence because for many people, families are the primary unit of interaction up until around that point. Once junior high hits, many young people begin to identify more effectively with their peer group than they do with family, and they actually begin to rebel against certain family values, which may include diet.

In addition, there are particularly hateful and obnoxious interactions with fellow seventh graders with regard to people who look different or act differently, particularly related to weight, in which negative and hateful patterns can develop. This section will begin to look at how friends and work colleagues may interfere with effective eating patterns.

Also, again in this exercise, note that things may have changed over the course of time. One example might be if you have a coworker colleague and the two of you have evolved into going out to lunch and eating particularly bad foods together on a regular basis. There may be resistance should you start to eat more healthful foods when your friend is not interested in the change. Be ready and prepared to deal with that.

EXPERIENCE #10: MIND MAP FRIENDS

Allow yourself a moment of silence and quietly ask yourself: Who is the most important person in my past, not a family member but a friend or perhaps even a bully or some other person, who influenced my eating patterns and my concept of weight and self? Allow the first impression to enter your awareness and write down the name of that person and their relationship to you in the middle of the mind map. Create a mind map based upon the question categories in this example specific to you.

Repeat this exercise with anyone else who comes to mind, asking the question. Again, these might include friends, colleagues, coworkers, enemies, bullies, perhaps even comments from television – anything you would consider related to relationships outside of the immediate family.

Again, after you have completed this set of mind maps, review them for common elements: common feelings, common themes, or for particular periods of time in life that led you to be more vulnerable to eating and document those similarities on a separate piece of paper. You can put that with the paper from the previous chapter and the next two chapters, and we will be working on those particular negative patterns later.

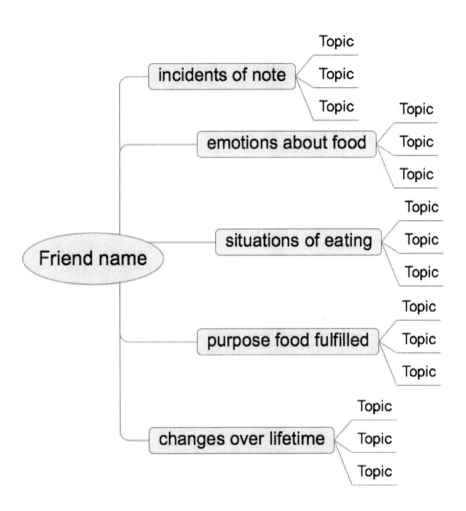

Chapter Eleven

Patterns of Situations

In this section, we are going to mind map situations that tend to lead to out-of-control eating behaviors. Rather than people, this will relate to settings, locations or events.

A key challenge that I find in Las Vegas is the endless array of giant buffets. I do not believe this is a challenge singular to me. There is an innate quality within all of us which would lead us to overeat in situations where there is an endless supply of food, especially in the context of having paid to enter the buffet and wanting to get money's worth for such.

For other people, particular challenges may be birthday parties, family events, holidays, or long weekends where we often give ourselves permission to be more free in eating patterns than we typically would during the average work week.

Also note as in the previous two chapters, these behaviors may have changed or altered over the course of time or may have been particularly affected by one or more particular life events, so when you make notations in these mind maps, also note if there were events that led changes to occur.

EXPERIENCE #11: MIND MAP SITUATIONS

Allow yourself a moment of silence and quietly ask yourself: What the most important situation is in my past that influenced my eating patterns and my concept of weight and self? Allow the first impression to enter your awareness and write down the situation and your role in that situation in the center of the mind map.

Create the rest of the mind map based upon the categories listed in the first branches, and add as many subbranches as you need to fully detail situations.

As is typical for mind maps, use minimal numbers of words but give enough words so that the entire experience will come back vividly when you just see those. Also, as with our other mind map exercises, feel free to add pictures, diagrams, drawings, or anything else that will make it more real for you.

When you have completed the first mind map in this sequence, repeat the exercise with each experience that saliently affected your eating, eating patterns, concept of weight, or concept of self, regarding weight.

When you have completed a set of these, put them together and review them. Again, make a list of the points which are common to these mind maps and include it with the list from the two previous chapters.

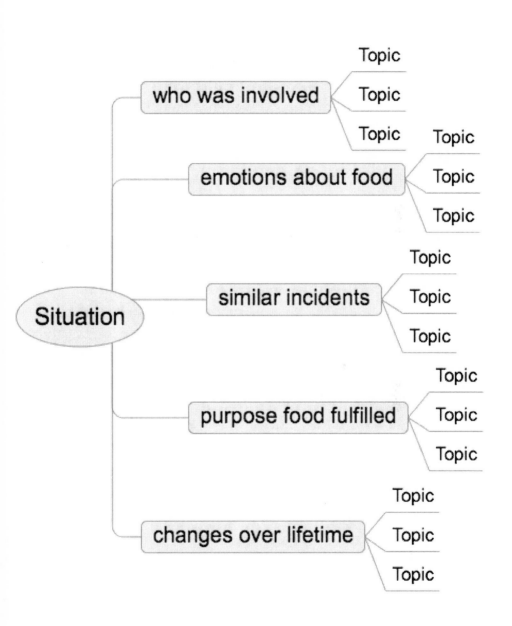

BEHAVIOR TIP #5: WAIT 20 MINUTES AFTER EATING A PORTION PRIOR TO EATING ANY MORE FOOD

This is an important exercise to develop. It will first allow you to enjoy and savor your meals more fully because you will not be as rushed to finish them, but more importantly, the innervation of the stomach takes a certain amount of time to fully communicate to the brain that it is now full and that it has adequate food within it to be satisfied.

A very clear example of this came up for me as recently as last week. I ate a very small salad over a hurried lunch with about two ounces of meat on the side, and when I finished eating the salad, I looked at it and said to myself, "Surely that was not enough. I ought to get some more of that to be full," but I got distracted by other things for a few minutes, and at the end of about twenty minutes, all of the feelings of hunger had dissipated and I no longer felt like I needed any more food.

I could have had more of the salad. It was on my diet and it was certainly appropriate and would not have taken me over my total calories for the day, but the point was by waiting for the twenty-minute mark, I did not feel like I even wanted the salad, or anything, for that matter, any longer.

This tip allows you to reduce the amount of food you are eating by allowing the signals to reach your brain to communicate that you are actually full.

Chapter Twelve

Patterns of Feelings

Not only do family, friends, past patterns, and situations drive eating, but for many of us, emotions drive eating as well. Some of us tend to eat if we are happy, some when we are sad to fill the depression and the emptiness, some when we are anxious to make the anxiety go away. Some people eat when they are angry and furious, and others of us eat no matter what our feeling is, but because eating changes the feeling into something different.

Also, many eat to attempt to avoid feeling whatsoever, as eating is a generally pleasurable activity and releases positive chemicals in the brain which relate to satiety. In this chapter, we are going to explore and discover this aspect of our food history.

Again, as in the two previous chapters, these feelings and concepts may have changed over the course of a life and may be the result of a particular event. If so, note that event carefully so that we can deal with it in one of the later chapters.

EXPERIENCE #12: MIND MAP FEELINGS

Allow yourself a moment of silence and quietly ask yourself what feelings in your past influenced your eating patterns and your concept of weight and self. Allow the first impression to enter your awareness and write it down – specifically the feeling, but also the situation which led to the feeling for the first time that you can recall -- in the middle of the mind map.

Create the balance of the mind map based upon the questions in the primary branches around the mind map by filling in the final branches in a manner specific to you.

When you have completed the first mind map, go back to the exercise and create additional mind maps for other feelings which actually affect your eating behavior. When you have completed a set of the mind maps and nothing else immediately comes to mind, review them as a group and identify any commonalities. Again, document that on a separate sheet of paper, and we will deal with this in a future chapter.

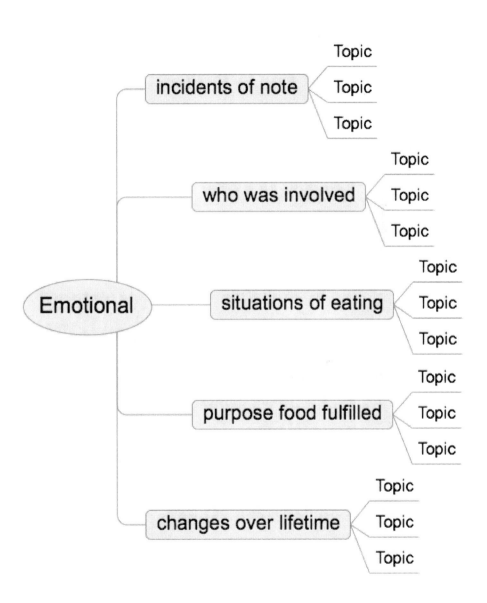

Chapter Thirteen

But I Want It!

Desire and Deprivation

One of the most pernicious patterns that develops over the course of time, both within a diet and after a diet, is a growing sense of dissatisfaction combined with an internal sense of deeply wanting a particular food. The sense of deprivation follows and intensifies each time you decline the food choice, until despair causes a failure in the diet.

The first few attempts in this cycle, willpower suffices as a means of dealing with saying no, but after several rounds, willpower will fail for the reasons that we discussed earlier, and the sense of deprivation of _Why do I have to give this up when my friend does not?_ begins to insidiously take over. Eventually willpower caves and the difficult food wins.

This is a powerful set of emotions, and I believe it underlies many of the failures at some point along the diet path. The simplest counter to the cycle is to attempt a food substitution. Some of these food substitutions are quite easily accomplished and eliminate the notion of deprivation altogether. Other food substitutions are less effective and will require further action.

An example of a food substitution might be something along the lines of trading a regular chocolate bar for either a low-carbohydrate chocolate bar or a low-fat chocolate bar, depending upon which diet you follow. If the taste of your substitute is adequate to the food you are replacing, often the deprivation cycle will automatically be short-circuited at that very point, and you will have found an acceptable alternative.

This is the optimal outcome within this cycle because it is easily accomplished and requires little effort. However, if this is not successful, you can continue with the next step.

Antidote

Identify the feeling that you experience with the food that you are deeply desiring to have but know would not be in your best interest. If you are in the middle of a restaurant when this is occurring, scribble down some information or put a note in your smart phone to deal with it more thoroughly at a later point.

When you have the time, examine that feeling and ask yourself, "Is it honestly true that I am deprived because I cannot eat food X?"

What is driving this feeling if not true deprivation? Beginning to untangle the sense of deprivation from some of the other emotional states that may be driving the food is important because deprivation is hard to deal with directly. If you find out, however, that you are frustrated as opposed to feeling deprived, you may be able to fulfill the frustration in another manner.

If you are feeling like it is generally unfair because your best friend can eat the chocolate cake and you cannot, then you can begin to look at whether it is reasonable to feel unfair with your friend as opposed to dealing directly with the chocolate cake matter. Dealing with these attendant feelings can then free you to make other food choices without having these negative other feelings clinging to your decision and attached.

If, however, you eventually decide none of those other feelings apply, none of anything else applies - you are simply feeling deprived, you must have it or life will be incomplete – then eat a single bite of the food, chew it as slowly as possible and genuinely, honestly, thoroughly and completely savor the taste of that bite totally without guilt, and then push the rest of the plate away.

After you push it away, tell yourself with as strong a mental voice as you can muster that at any time your feeling of deprivation reaches a crisis level, you can have another bite of this food. It is not gone forever and it is not something that must be completely eliminated forever. This will give you a greater sense of control and allow you to loosen up the tightness with which the deprivation cycle can hold you.

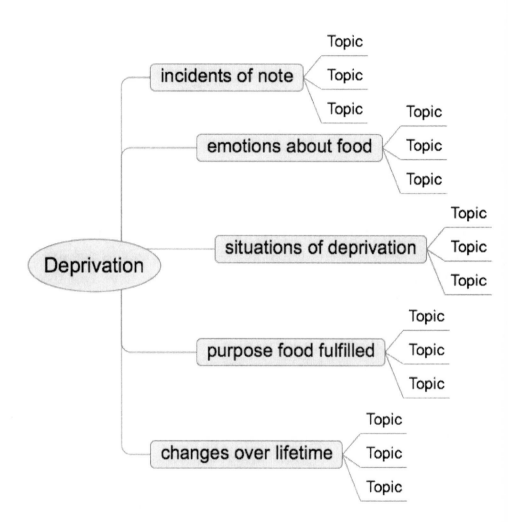

BEHAVIOR TIP # 6: EAT ALL THE SALAD YOU WANT

There is almost no food that could not be mixed with salad, and salad has very few calories, virtually no fat and virtually no carbohydrates. You can eat lettuce and other green leafy vegetables on virtually any diet.

The only difference is if you are on a low-carbohydrate diet, you would choose blue cheese dressing or Caesar dressing typically, and if you are on a low-fat diet, you would probably choose something like balsamic vinaigrette with no oil, but the lettuce itself can be eaten almost in unlimited supplies. It will help you fill up such that you do not feel hungry or deprived, and if you have a piece of meat or tofu or other kinds of protein, you can add it to the salad and have a full meal that is filling and complete.

EXPERIENCE #13: MIND MAP DEPRIVATION

Allow yourself a moment of silence and quietly ask yourself what the most recent experience was in which you felt deprived because of your food choices. Allow the first impression to enter awareness and write down the situation and your role within it in the center of the mind map.

Create the balance of the mind map based upon the earlier mind maps completed so far. Make this as specific to you and to your situation as possible.

Repeat this exercise with each situation that comes to mind, review the situations for areas in common and then make a list of commonalities. Place that on a piece of paper with the ones from the previous chapters, and we will use these examples in future exercises.

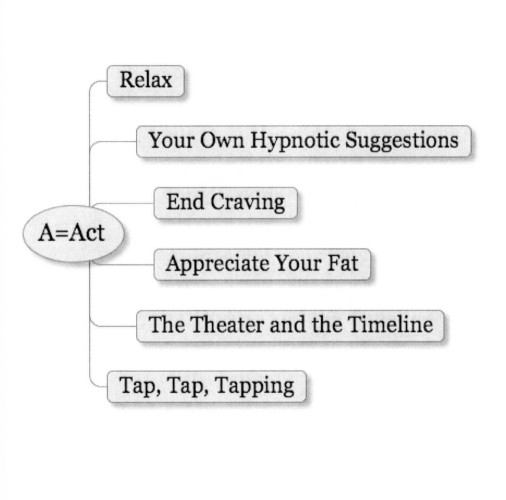

Chapter Fourteen

Relax

One of the most common emotional drives to eat has to do with feeling stressed or anxious, and many people eat in order to reduce emotion.

I will provide several different methods in this chapter to learn in relaxation exercises. Some of these will be also provided online in free audio files if you would like to download them from the website. www.newmindnewbody.com. Feel also free to make your own audio tape or audio file by reading these scripts into a digital recorder and then play them back for yourself.

EXPERIENCE #14: PROGRESSIVE RELAXATION

The progressive relaxation response was discovered by Dr. Herbert Benson in the 1960s and 1970s when medicine began to first identify the possibility that emotional states could affect such physiological measures as blood pressure. Dr. Benson developed a simple method, easy to follow, which I will paraphrase here.

Find a comfortable place on a chair. You can either sit or lie down for this exercise, but have time where you will not be interrupted by a telephone, a doorbell, or noise, especially the television. You will probably prefer to close your eyes through-out.

•Once you have sat down and gotten situated, tight-en all of the muscles in your feet as tightly as possible and particularly focus your attention on the muscle tension in those muscle groups.

•Once you have fully felt the muscle tension there, allow the muscles of your feet to completely relax. Pay close attention and notice the difference in feeling between the tight muscle and the loose, limp, relaxed muscle. You may have a sense of warmness, a sense of coolness, a sense of looseness. It will be individual to you, but have the ability to identify the difference in those two feelings.

•Next, tighten and clench all of the muscles in your calves and lower legs. Again, after you feel the ten-sion fully and experience it, let it go, let it melt away and then notice the feeling that arises once you have completely relaxed that muscle group.

•Once you have noticed that feeling clearly, then tense all of the muscles in your thighs and upper legs as tightly as possible, feel the tension there, and again relax, let the muscles go loose, limp, and easy.

•Continuing, tighten the muscles in your buttocks, lower back, and abdomen as tightly as you can, feel the muscle tension in those muscle groups. Once you have a good feeling of all of those muscle groups being tight, allow them to completely relax and go loose and limp. Notice the difference in conscious awareness between the tension and the relaxation. Identify that feeling so that you can notice it in the future.

•Next, tighten and clench the muscles in your hands as tightly as possibly. Notice the tension. Allow the tension to go when you release your muscles and notice the difference.

•Clench the muscles in your lower arms and upper arms. Notice the tightness, notice the tension, feel and appreciate it, and then allow them to go loose, limp, and relaxed and notice the difference with the feeling of relaxation in comparison with the feeling of tension.

•Next, tighten all the muscles in your upper back, shoulders, and neck. This area of the body tends to carry a lot of tension anyway, but accentuate that tension by tightening the muscles. Again, after you have tightened them, allow them to go completely relaxed, loose, and limp, and notice the difference in the feeling in these particular muscle groups.

•You may want to repeat this exercise with your neck and upper shoulders just because of the extra tension often stored there.

•Next, tighten the muscles of your face, mouth, and

around the eyes and jaw as tightly as you can, also the top of your head and scalp, and after you feel the tension there, let it go loose, limp, and relaxed. You will find that your entire body has a lesser degree of muscle tension after completing this sequence.

•It is now possible to imagine, in whatever way you like, a wave of relaxing energy starting at your feet and moving up through your body with a warmth or a coolness, whichever you prefer, and allow it to move from the bottom of your feet to the top of your head.

•Scan your body now and see if there is any body part that still feels tight, tense, or uncomfortable. If so, send another wave of relaxation through your body and focus it on that particular area. Repeat until that area feels as relaxed as the surrounding regions.

•Take a few minutes to just relax in this state, and after you feel complete, open your eyes and rejoin the world.

This exercise trains the parasympathetic nervous system to begin to counteract the overactivity of the sympathetic nervous system. The sympathetic nervous system mediates stress and anxiety, and the flight/fight response. The parasympathetic nervous system balances that out. It aids in digestion, it aids in relaxation, and it reduces anxiety and stress.

Regular practice of this type of relaxation exercise can help you deal with stressful situations with less subjective sensations of stressfulness. I would note, however, you need to practice it on a regular basis, not just at those times you feel stressed, because if you try to practice it when you are already feeling stressed, you will get less robust effects than if you have already mastered the technique in less stressful situations.

BEHAVIOR TIP #7: SAVOR YOUR FOOD AND NOTICE HOW IT CHANGES

Take a few moments during your next meal and notice that the first bite of a particularly wonderful piece of food tastes awesome, but then each bite that follows, although it may taste good, tastes less awesome than the first bite tasted.

If you observe this over the course of meals and the course of different foods, you will begin to notice that five or six bites into most entrees, the food does not have that magically wonderful feeling that it did when you first started eating it. At that point, consider that you may have eaten all of that particular food that you need to eat.

There is a particular dessert at Texas De Brazil steakhouse that is truly beyond wonderful to me. The Bananas Foster Pie contains a combination of flavors that on the first bite resembles true ecstasy. The next bites, though, lessen in intensity. If I'm going to stray from my usual food choice, one bite of this amazing dessert is my limit, because I am aware that the first bite is by far the best.

The key component of this particular behavioral tip is to

truly enjoy the food as you are eating it and to not wolf it down and finish it in the quickest possible manner.

EXPERIENCE #15: THE SIMPLEST MEDITATON OF ALL

Everyone breathes. You can use this meditation without any additional technology. All you need to do is sit down and begin to focus your awareness on your breath. Each time you breathe in, say to yourself, "The breath flows in," and each time you breathe out, say to yourself, "The breath flows out."

Continue to repeat this for approximately ten minutes and try to work up closer to twenty minutes. Observe your emotional state before you start this exercise and after you finish the exercise.

One of the issues with the progressive relaxation technique earlier in this chapter is that often after the body becomes fully relaxed, the mind actually has a number of items racing through it, such as *What is my next meal going to be?* or *Where do I need to be at 2:00 this afternoon?* or *I have a telephone call scheduled; am I going to finish this in time?*

Relaxing the body without relaxing the mind is less helpful than the capacity to relax both together. This exercise complements and finishes the first exercise because this focus on your breathing allows you to relax and focus your mind in a clear manner that keeps those external thoughts out.

Invariably after five or ten or fifteen breaths, thinking

nothing other than *the breath flows in* and *the breath flows out*, suddenly those very same distracting thoughts will start to leap into your mind as if they are important. This is okay. Do not get distraught. Simply become aware of those thoughts as they interrupt you, and then bring your focus back to your assigned task, which is to focus on *the breath flows in, the breath flows out.*

Expect mental interruption. This is not a problem with your technique; it is the way that our minds work, but you can refocus on the meditation for the period of time that you have set aside for yourself.

EXPERIENCE #16: THOUGHT-AS-BUBBLES MEDITATION

Earlier, I mentioned that it is useful to begin to observe thoughts and feelings as if they were in a third-person state, or not directly part of you, so that you can look at them without being quite so intensely focused upon them. This meditation is ideal for this purpose and allows you to practice in a neutral state with emotions that probably are not terribly distracting.

- Again, sit down and make yourself comfortable, and this time allow whatever comes to mind to come to mind but simply roll it into a bubble and let it float out of awareness as soon as it enters your mind.

- You can envision this as being something like a fish tank where each thought that arises turns into a bubble and floats up to the top to disappear. If this is a disturbing thought or problematic thought, awesome. Turn it into a bubble and let it float to the top and disappear. If it is a bored thought, great. Turn it into a bubble and let it float to the top and disappear.

•Just be aware these are thoughts and they are disappearing and floating away. They are not you; they simply are thoughts, mental contents, or feelings.

•Let us say that your mind decides to rebel against this practice, and you have no thought whatsoever but simply blackness in mental awareness. This is absolutely fantastic because the blackness is also a thought, so simply roll the blackness into a bubble and let it float away as well. Eventually another thought content will arrive, and you will begin to continue with the meditation.

Observe your emotions and your bodily state both before and after you practice this experience and begin to appreciate the capacity to look at your inner thoughts as if they are bubbles floating away rather than something that you have to deal with in the immediate time here and now.

Binaural Beat Technology

Binaural beats were discovered by Dr. Heinrich Dove in the nineteenth century, and they are part of a biological mechanism in your brain that helps you locate things in space. For example, if you are in the middle of a field and hear some kind of a rustling noise over to your right, the sound wave that arrives at your right and your left ear will be slightly different because your right ear and your left ear are a slightly different distant from that sound.

Your brain immediately transfers this into information to allow you to turn your head to look directly at the location of the sound. This obviously had incredible survival mechanisms built into it, because if this was a wild beast in ancient days, you would have the opportunity to get away from it by localizing it through your hearing before you had to identify it only with vision, at which point it might be too late.

However, if two different sounds of very close quality are put into each ear and you cannot turn your head to localize something because there is nothing to localize, your brain will entrain to the difference in the two frequencies of sound.

As an example, if a 100-Hz sound is put in the left ear and a 104-Hz sound is put in the right ear, your brain will entrain to a 4-Hz pattern. This pattern relates to a lower rate of brain waves which is meditative and relaxing.

Without going into great detail about each of the brain wave states and how they may affect you in subjective experience, it will suffice to say that there are excellent products available which use binaural beat technology to effectively induce a highly relaxed state very quickly and one in which you can experience it passively without having to engage in active exercises as we did in the early exercises of this chapter.

One particular tape which is excellent for this is produced by the Monroe Institute, and it is called "Hemi-sync Meditation." It can be downloaded as an audio file from their website or purchased as a CD. You can use this technology to aid you in any of the exercises later in the book if you wish to be in a more relaxed state when doing the exercises. 7Or, you can use the earlier techniques from this chapter.

Self-hypnosis

Many people say that they believe they cannot be hypnotized, and for a very tiny minority of people, that could perhaps be true. However, if you have ever had the experience of driving down the highway in a car and lost track of time, realizing that ten or fifteen minutes perhaps have passed since you were really consciously aware of sitting in the car, or if you have sat in a movie theater and gotten lost in the action of a movie and suddenly look at your watch and realize half an hour has gone by in the movie, you have in fact been in a light state of hypnosis.

Hypnosis is a normal state of mind and a normal state of functioning, and we enter it on a relatively regular basis.

As noted earlier, Milton Erickson suggested that we are always in a state of hypnosis which is why advertising and politicians are so effective in affecting our emotional states and buying habits. However, irrespective, any form of hypnosis is essentially consensual to a large degree, and even when you see a staged hypnosis show with people doing outrageous things in public, they have consented to do so and they do not have any major objection to the actions they have been asked to perform, so all hypnosis, at least at some level, is a form of self-hypnosis.

The benefit of this state, as we discussed in the chapter on the hypnotic model of the mind, is that the combination of physical relaxation with the particular mental state defined as somnambulism allows for the entry of new material into the unconscious which will effectively skip over the gatekeeper.

It is most likely the case when you experience hypnosis for the first time that you will believe you are in fact not hypnotized because, subjectively, you may experience very little different than what you experience in waking states other than perhaps being slightly more relaxed, but you will not necessarily notice a huge mental difference, especially the first few times that you experience it.

In the next experience, I am going to share with you the Elman rapid induction for hypnosis and will include several additional suggestions to allow you to reach the state more easily and more deeply whenever you wish to in the future. You will likely need to create or download an audio copy of this. This is a variant of the original induction altered to allow for use without the hypnotist being personally present.

There are a remarkably tiny number of individuals who can become anxious when they enter into any kind of meditative, relaxed, or hypnotic state. If you have had any problems in the first exercises of this chapter in achieving a relaxed state or you find when you attempt to relax you begin to feel markedly more anxious, this is a sign that you probably should not go through the hypnotic exercise but should rather go and see a professional before engaging a hypnotic routine, as you could be an individual who could become quite anxious during the experience. If you do become markedly anxious, open your eyes and repeat to yourself that the experience is fading, ground by eating or engaging in physical activity.

EXPERIENCE #17: THE ELMAN RAPID INDUCTION

This variant of the Elman induction is one possible to accomplish without the hypnotist physically present. In addition, I have included some basic deepening material to help you gain control over the practice of entering into deeper states of hypnosis.

The key mental attitude to approach this experience with is the attitude of play and fun. There is a section, for example, that will tell you to test whether you are actually relaxed by testing whether you can open your eyelids. You can, of course, prove to yourself that you are not relaxed by opening your eyelids, but all you have done is to prove what you already knew, that you could, in fact, open your eyelids. If you want to experience what the experience has to offer, play along with experiencing what it would be like for your eyelids to feel so heavy that you cannot open them, and you will get there. Prove to yourself that for a few minutes you can't open you eyelids and see what it is like.

•Take a long, deep breath, fill your lungs up really well and hold it for a second. Now when you exhale, close your eyes down and let yourself relax. Get rid of that surface tension in your body. Let your shoulders relax, let your body relax. It is okay to relax now.

•Now put your awareness on your eyelids. Know that you can relax those eyes beautifully. You know that you can relax those eyes so deeply that as long as you choose not to remove that relaxation, your eyelids just will not work, and when you know you have done that, hold on to that relaxation.

•Give it a good test. Make sure they will not work and notice how good it feels. Test them hard. That is good. Stop testing and let yourself relax even more.

•Now let us really deepen this state.

•In a moment, I will ask you to open and close your eyes. When you close your eyes, send a wave of relaxation through your body so very quickly you would allow this physical part of you to relax ten times deeper. Just want it and you can have it.

•Let your eyes become open, close your eyes and really, really, really let go. Feel your body relax much more. You are doing fine. In a moment, I will ask you to open and close your eyes again.

•This time, when you close your eyes, double the physical relaxation. Let it go twice as deep. Let your eyes become down, way down, deeper, deeper, relaxed.

•In a moment, we will do it one more time and notice how well it comes in this time as you learn how simple it is. At least double it.

•Let your eyes open, way down, close, deeper, deeper, deeper.

•Can you feel that increase in relaxation? You should be able to feel that increase in relaxation all through your body. This is physical relaxation, and if you followed my instructions exactly, you should have an excellent state of physical relaxation this very minute, but we want to increase this relaxation even more.

•There are two ways in which you can relax: You can relax physically and you can relax mentally. You have proven that you can relax physically, now let us relax mentally. Here is how.

•In a moment, I want you to start counting backwards from 100 with me, silently in your mind with the idea that you are going to relax the numbers right out of your mind. In other words, you are going to let those numbers go by commanding your mind to relax as you count.

• In a moment, I want you to start from 100 and count back with me mentally so that when you get to 98, you will find that all of a sudden all the numbers after 98 will have completely disappeared.

• Now say the first number with me silently and relax as you do so:

• 100. That is right. Now relax completely, and when the next number comes up, they will begin to fade as you order them to leave your mind.

• 99. Get rid of those numbers. Just say to yourself they must disappear, and as you relax mentally, they will disappear and you will feel a surge of relaxation.

• Now say the last number: 98, and they will be gone. You just cannot find any numbers anywhere.

• This is what is known a complete physical and mental relaxation. If for any reason the numbers have not disappeared, do not worry. They will leave as I continue to talk with you.

• This ends the formal Elman induction, but we will now continue with the deepening technique to allow you to reach this state more easily each time you wish to practice in the future.

• Imagine, if you will, a stairwell or an elevator, which-ever is more comfortable for you, and we are going to count down. With each step down, you will feel more relaxed, more comfortable and more at ease.

• Ten – deeper and deeper.

• Nine – more relaxed, letting everything and every concern go.

• Eight . . .

• Seven . . . deeper and deeper.

• Six . . .

• Five . . . complete and total relaxation.

• Four . . .

• Three . . .

• Two . . .

• And one.

• Any sounds that you may hear from the outside, the hallways, you can choose to transform those sounds into yet more deep relaxation experiences, deeper and deeper with every sound you hear, more relaxed, more content, more focused.

•Know that you can return to this peaceful state of complete relaxation any time you want in the future and know that each time you return to this state, it will be deeper and easier than it ever has in the past.

•Take a few moments, enjoy this, and then I will count you back out to usual waking consciousness. In a moment, I am going to count to three, and when I reach the number three, you will be back in your usual alert, awake, mentally clear state.

•Number one . . . begin to notice the chair that is holding you up and begin to become aware of the room that you are sitting in.

•Number two . . . beginning to get clearer, noticing that when I reach the number one, you will be perfectly clear, alert, excellent, focused, and healthier in every way.

•Number three . . . open your eyes, awake, clear, awake.

Chapter Fifteen

Your Own Hypnotic Suggestions

The way to use the state that we just experienced after the Elman induction is to begin to create suggestions that are specific to you so that you can begin to insert new thoughts and ideas into your unconscious mind when in that state you are able to bypass the guardian or the gatekeeper which keeps the positive information out.

How to Use a Hypnotic Suggestion

There are two main ways that you can use this with a hypnotic suggestion yourself. The first is to read the entire sequence, but in the midst of it after the deepening exercise, simply add in a series of ten or twelve suggestions, either the same or different, that you have written for yourself, before the count out. This allows you to create your own tape that you can listen to any time you want. It is easy to accomplish either with a digital recorder or using software, such as GarageBand.

If you do not want to make your own tape and you want to use the audio already created on the website, you can simply tell yourself the suggestions that you have written immediately before the exercise and repeat them immediately after the exercise. You will have a window of approximately thirty seconds after the count of three at the end of the wakeup to continue to add material that will be accepted in the unconscious.

In the first thirty seconds after completing the web version, simply read the hypnotic suggestions that you have written for yourself in that thirty seconds as many times as you can fit into the thirty seconds.

How to Write a Hypnotic Suggestion

If you are going to be speaking a hypnotic suggestion to yourself live, then use the word "I," such as, "I am healthy and at a perfect weight."

If you are going to be taping them and playing the tape back to yourself, use the word "you," because you will be listening to a tape and you will want to hear the words, "*you* choose to eat healthily, happily, and maintain a perfect weight."
Second, use the present verb tense. If you give the unconscious a suggestion that is in the future, then it will remain in the future.

As an example, if you write a suggestion that says, "I want to be thin." Your unconscious will interpret this to mean not that you plan to actually *be* thin but rather that you *want* to be thin, so you can remain quite heavy and still *want* to be thin. The suggestion worked absolutely perfectly because you want to be thin, perhaps with more intensity than you ever had before. So carefully word the suggestions so that they mean exactly what you want them to mean.

The next point is to avoid or eliminate all negative terms

in your suggestion. The unconscious does not typically understand or process the word, "no." This phenomenon is called, "pharsing" in hypnotic circles, and I will provide you an amusing example of what happened to me.

I made a type of hypnotic suggestion in which the suggestion was, "I will lose five pounds in the next two weeks," and I used this for several days in a row, and two weeks later when I stepped on the scale, the scale was exactly five pounds different, but it was five pounds up because the word, "lose" is a negative word that my unconscious could not appropriately process.

Instead of saying you want to lose a certain amount of weight, instead you want to suggest what your perfect weight might be. For example, *My perfect weight is blank, and I weigh blank.* Repeat that phrase as a hypnotic suggestion, and it will begin to enter your unconscious. Note that it is in the present tense, and it does not use a negative, it only uses a positive.

Examples of Hypnotic Suggestions

I am in vibrant health.

My food choices create the body I desire.

I eat only when I feel physically hungry.

I am attracted to the foods perfect for me and my diet.

I value my health.

Exercise is easy for me.

I exercise daily without exception.

I love and accept my perfect body.

My perfect weight is _____ AND I am at my perfect weight.

EXPERIENCE #18: WRITE YOUR OWN HYPNOTIC SUGGESTIONS

Using the ideas above combined with your particular weight goals and your particular plans, write at least ten hypnotic suggestions for yourself. Use these daily for the next few weeks and monitor your progress. However, do not use all ten the same day. Pick one suggestion and use it for several days then switch to the next one, use it for several days, and continue in this sequence.

Make notes in the days after you have used a particular suggestion whether or not you have a different perception about food, different impulses towards eating, or any changes in the positive direction that you seek. When you see this, it is a particularly good hypnotic suggestion that you have written for yourself. You can repeat it and fashion other hypnotic suggestions in a similar manner.

BEHAVIOR TIP #8: WHEN YOU HAVE A CRAVING TO EAT OR WHEN YOU SIT DOWN AT A TABLE TO EAT, SIT DOWN FOR A FEW MINUTES AND ASK YOURSELF, "AM I ACTUALLY HUNGRY RIGHT NOW?"

If the answer to yourself is yes, awesome, eat; but if the answer is no, ask yourself, "What is pushing me to desire to eat right now since it is not hunger? Is it an emotion, place, person, or thing?"

When something comes to mind, ask yourself, "What could satisfy this other than eating right now?"

This exercise will allow you to begin to determine whether or not you are eating for the purpose of hunger, which is a reasonable reason to eat, or whether you are eating for the purpose of fulfilling another need, in which case this allows you the opportunity to view the situation from a third-party perspective, much as the thoughts in the bubble, and to see it as if it is not immediately happening to you now.

It puts in a stop mechanism so that you can choose to do something else rather than automatically following through on the eating behavior.

Chapter Sixteen

End Craving

One of the offshoots from the hypnosis system of Dr. Milton Erickson discussed earlier is a system called neurolinguistic programming (NLP). NLP has been used so successfully in marketing that to seriously question its validity is folly. It builds upon the model of the hypnotic mind to provide other techniques to get material past the gatekeeper, often with little conscious awareness.

One of the aspects of NLP is the concept that various pieces of information are stored experientially in the brain, specifically, this would be occurring in the association network. Some NLP techniques can aid in removing the associations that attach to the reward centers as we discussed earlier in the book. One of the powerful techniques for ending craving is the capacity to experience how you are storing the mental contents of a particular activity or thing. You can actually use this technique for other things that come up if you wish, but it is particularly useful for dealing with problem foods.

I will give a brief description here and then give a script for you to follow as part of an experience.

When we mentally represent something, we can either represent it in an auditory manner, a visual manner, a kinesthetic manner, or occasionally an auditory digital manner. All of us are different in this respect, and we all draw these pieces of information of our lives together in one or more of these types of processing, typically called, "modalities" by NLP practitioners.

A particular food that you love is going to be stored in particular ways in one or more of these modalities, and you can compare and contrast how you are storing the food you love and crave with a food that you find disgusting and horrific because they have to be stored in at least a slightly different way or you would perceive them both as being wonderful foods. With that as a background, we will move on to the technique itself.

EXPERIENCE #19: END CRAVING NOW

Sit down in a quiet space where you are unlikely to be interrupted and make yourself comfortable. You can use one of the relaxation techniques from an earlier chapter or put on a CD that you find particularly relaxing, likely a binaural beat program as opposed to music, but something that will allow you to be mentally quiet and focused so that you can follow through with the exercise.

Next, bring to mind the food that is problematic and that you crave with a craving that just will not let go. Experience the mental representation of this food. This may be a bodily sensation, it may be a physical picture of the food in front of your eyes, it may be a verbal statement or a verbal commentary about the food that is almost auditory in nature. It does not matter. Just bring a representation to your awareness.

Notice through all of the exercises, I use the word, "imagine," not the word, "visualize," because you can bring this into your imagination in any manner you like.

This particular script is going to use a visual metaphor; however, you can modify the script if you are experiencing it in an auditory manner or in a tactile manner. It does not matter, but get the notion of what the script is trying to do.

After you have experienced this, begin asking yourself a series of questions. If it is in the visual realm, you will ask: Was the picture of this food in color or in black and white? Does it have a frame around it or is it unframed? Is it in the center of your vision, right, left, up, down? Where do you see it happening, if you are seeing it? Is it blurry or clear? Does it have other items around it, or is it by itself? Is it large or is it small?

Next, let this image of the craved food fade from your mind and make a note of each one of those questions. If there is anything else notable about what is happening, write that down as well. Alter the question set if you experience the food representation in a nonvisual way.

After you have cleared your mind from this food that you craved, now bring into your mind the most revolting, disgusting food that you can imagine. If you cannot imagine a revolting or disgusting food because it all seems so awesome, then bring something nonedible that is disgusting to mind, like a drain full of hair and rotting material – it does not matter as long as you find it gross.

Then close your eyes and bring that into your awareness as well and ask again the same questions. Very typically, the answers will be different. One of them will be in color, another one will be in black and white. One of them will be in the left lower part of your vision; the other will be in the center, just as examples. Note each one of those qualities in this particular mental representation of something utterly reprehensible.

Make check marks next to the things that are different on your two lists. As an example, if your favorite food that you crave is in the center of your vision and in vivid color and the disgusting food is on the lower left part of your vision in black and white, and those are the two differences between the two, note what they are.

Now close your eyes again, bring up the visual representation of the craved food and drag it down into the area of the disgusting food, shrinking it and turning it into black and white at the same time.

After you have done this, reassess your interest in the food that you were craving several moments ago. If you had an auditory experience rather than a visual experience, ask yourself the quality of the auditory experience, the type of experience. Was it a voice? Was it a sensation? Was it a hum?

If you had a tactile sensation, where was it? How big was

it? Was it pleasant or unpleasant? Where was it on your body? Did it have a color? Use that modality to switch the craved food into the reprehensible food location or placement. It will work the same in the nonvisual medium.

If there is another food which you also have an intense craving for, follow the same exercise using the second food, and continue this process until the main foods of craving have been eliminated as cravings.

Chapter Seventeen

Appreciate Your Fat

Every part of us is important to who we have been and who we have become, and every part has formed some form of a purpose for all of this time, whether we are aware of it or not, whether we like it or not and whether we hate it or not.

Fat is an integral part of our identity, and how we have carried it is part of who we are and who we appear to be. If there is any question, just notice the responses from other people at a class reunion when people have lost or gained large amounts of weight and how they respond to each other.

This is perhaps one of the more painful or probing exercises in the book because people tend to assume that fat is negative and has served no purpose for them. This leads to a demonization of the fat itself, and the intense emotions that go along with that may trap the fat into being present because whether we like something or we hate something, we are deeply attached to it in one way or another. Review the chapter on blame and reframe the comments on blame into comments on hate.

Working through this internal dichotomy is not necessarily difficult, but it does take a little bit of focus.

EXPERIENCE #20: MIND MAP THE BENEFITS OF BEING OVERWEIGHT

Yes, you heard me: The *benefits* of being overweight. Lest ye be unaware that there are benefits, for the first forty-nine years of my life, I was hot everywhere that I ever went and needed the air conditioning on. After losing sixty pounds, I am now freezing everywhere I go and cannot bear cold air. It is an entirely new experience for me. Having to carry a sweater around in the middle of the summer is not a plus.

Take a few moments of quiet and create a mind map whose central core is the benefit provided by your weight and your fat. The focus of this mind map is to look at each and every way that being overweight has been a benefit to you psychologically or physically. No negatives on this. This may be a deeply emotional exercise, and that is okay. Take your time with it.

Love Conquers All

Love, very much like consciousness, is accepting, inclusive, and without judgment. Appreciating your weight for the purpose it served you in the past is an amazing healing activity; whereas, holding on to hate or anger towards weight, much like blame, only makes you attached to it and a victim of it.

In many situations, weight acts as an insulation against deeper feelings and also may act as an insulation against others. It may have helped us stay away from others in the past because we were afraid of being hurt by them, and so putting a layer of insulation between them and us felt like a very positive and supportive thing to do.

Some individuals who have had the terrible misfortune of being assaulted, either physically or sexually, may gain substantial amounts of weight to attempt to make themselves look unattractive to feel personally safer; whereas, in fact the evildoing on the part of the perpetrator was not motivated typically by attraction in the first place, but by aggression.

Using the above mind map, characterize the benefits of the weight and what it has given you up until this point in life, and then we will move forward into the next experience.

EXPERIENCE #21: THE PARTS EXERCISE

Close your eyes, take a few moments of quiet and relax peacefully. Again, you can use a relaxation exercise or a binaural beats technology tape to get yourself in a mentally focused, clear and relaxed state and imagine in one hand all of the things, experiences, and aspects of your weight and eating behavior that you dislike and ways that this has been a disservice to you and the reasons, to a degree, why you wish to lose the weight.

When you have some sense of this in whatever imaginable state you experience, open your other hand on the other side of your body and imagine there all of the benefits, help, ideas and genuine positive results that have resulted from the weight that you have carried to this point.

Once you have this information set and this feeling state symbolized in your two hands, ask yourself, "Is there a way that I can keep all of these positive things that my weight has done for me without having to carry all of this weight?"

Slowly allow the two hands to come together and allow them to come together and touch at the point you internally know that these two parts are now one, can work together, and can give you all of the benefits, help, and protection that the weight did without the health detriments, the discomfort, and the unpleasantness of the excess weight itself.

After you have clasped your hands together and collapsed these two polarities into one, thank yourself and thank your weight for all that it has done for you in the past, and let go. Express gratitude.

Chapter Eighteen

The Timeline and the Theater

There are many experiences that you have discovered in the course of making mind maps from situations, family, friends, and emotions that are caused by a particular event that occurred in the past that created the shape of your string, thereby leading to the pearls.

We are going to use two different techniques to help modify the string and eliminate the pearls, and these two exercises are the timeline exercise and the theater exercise. Feel free to use both of them and feel free to trade them back and forth because they accomplish similar ends, but you may be more comfortable with one versus the other. Both are variants of NLP style techniques.

Note that the synergy between the first pearl and the energetic string is high, so if you deal with the first episode of a problematic incident, it will probably help many of the rest of the pearls just disappear on their own and will help remake the string.

The problem is that this first pearl and the shape of your string upon which the pearls lie happened prior to you becoming consciously aware. Had you become consciously aware sooner, you probably would have helped form it in a more positive way, but many of these experiences happened in childhood or with traumas or simply negative experiences that occurred before you knew what was happening around you.

Then, much like a movie, this is played over and over again from the unconscious and repeats until it is changed, much as we discussed in an earlier chapter.

The move theater technique is designed to be gentle; however, it does replay certain instances from the past that you choose, under your control, and could, therefore, be stressful.

A metaphor I like to use to describe this, though, is the actors who participate in a gruesome horror movie. If you sit and watch the movie in the theater, you may be unnerved by the terrible things that are happening to people on the screen. And yet had you been there when the movie was filmed, once the director yelled, "Cut!" all the actors would jump up, smile and say, "What a great job we just did! That should really scare people."

The actors are not actually hurt in the scene, and anything that comes up for you in these exercises really no longer has the capacity to hurt you, because all of this may be an unpleasant movie, but it is something from the past that is long past, and the people involved cannot hurt you anymore. All of it is all you at this point in life.

If you can see this in a similar light as a repetitious movie that can no longer directly hurt you, it provides the resilience to go through the exercise should it get difficult. Again, it is designed to be gentle as it stands.

EXPERIENCE #22: THE MOVIE THEATER

Take a few moments. Find a comfortable place to sit so that you can relax, be centered. You may want to use a relaxation exercise again, but you want to be alert and able to follow. Look at the mind maps that you have generated over the course of this material so far and find a particular person, place, or event that was challenging to you, difficult to you or led to a pattern of negative behavior related to your eating.

• Imagine yourself sitting in a theater with a giant screen in front of you.

• After you have some imagination of this, now imagine yourself back in the projection booth not watching the movie but watching yourself in the front row of the theater watching the movie. You do not even have to see the content of the movie from where you are standing in the projection booth because you are just watching you, you are not watching the movie directly.

• Start the movie a few moments before the troubling event occurred and play it in very rapid motion to its conclusion. This should not take more than two seconds, no matter how long the event actually was.

•Now play it backward in black and white, forward again in color quickly, backward slowly in black and white and forward quickly in color.

•Notice when you are performing this act whether or not the event is giving you any kind of emotion or anxiety, and if it is, continue playing the event backward and forward until you do not experience any anxiety from your perception as the person in the movie booth watching you watching the movie.

•Once there is no emotional tone left in this experience, now move your awareness to the person sitting in the movie theater instead of the person in the projection booth and again let this event play forward and backward, forward and backward at varying speeds, sometimes in color, sometimes in black and white, and again monitor whether you experience any anxiety from this experience. If you do, continue playing it in these various permutations, backward and forward until you do not have an emotional reaction any longer.

•Once this is completed, simply address the you who was in the movie theater from your present awareness and consciousness and tell them one thing you would like them to know based upon your now more mature view of reality. For example, if the experience was as a young child where the child felt unloved, you as an adult might say, "You may not know it, but you are greatly loved if by no one other than me," and if you wish, you can then mentally give the child in that image a hug and tell them everything will be okay. Make some kind of interaction with that representation of you at the younger point in life.

•Once this feels complete to you, you can open your eyes and come back to your usual state of consciousness.

This exercise should have eliminated any negative emotional impressions from the experience that you identified as being problematic related to your eating.

You can use this exercise with any of the other experiences you have determined in your mind maps to eliminate the negative feelings associated with the memory of the event. Once the feeling state is eliminated from it, it will no longer drive your behavior, and that pearl will drop off your string forever. It also energetically reshapes the string a bit, so future pearls will be more positive.

EXPERIENCE #23: THE TIMELINE

We all tend to put our experiences on a mental representation of a timeline. You can very easily determine where your timeline is by closing your eyes and imagining simply a place in space where you were when you were brushing your teeth yesterday. Then again, imagine where you probably will be in two or three days brushing your teeth.

You will likely have a notion of past on the left, future on the right, or you will have a notion of past behind you and future in front of you. These are two different versions of a timeline experience. The timeline is metaphorical, but it relates to how you place events into your sense of time.

There are certain differences in the way people interact in the world depending on these particular timeline strategies; however, they will not make any difference with regard to this particular exercise.

Pick another one of the examples from a mind map of a troubling life experience.

Now sit down peacefully and comfortably again, go through a relaxation exercise and take yourself above your timeline. Imagine your timeline like a small road below you with all the events of your life, like little flickering lights, but take yourself high enough above the timeline so that you cannot see any of the experiences directly.

Now take yourself along the timeline and ask yourself, "When is the first experience of this painful event/emotion that led to this problem with eating," using the information from the mind map as a guide, and now keep yourself above the timeline, looking down at this event, which is very tiny and far below you. If the event is bringing an emotional tone, go higher above the timeline.

For an instant, note the feeling of the event, and note its

impact. Then return above the timeline again. Take yourself a few hours prior to this experience and ask yourself where the feeling is. The feeling that arose from the experience should be absent since the event will not have occurred yet in the timeline. Thank the event for the important information and allow the emotions to dissipate. This will neutralize the negative feeling that occurred during the experience.

Ask yourself if there are other experiences in the timeline that need to be neutralized, and if so, go to each one of them.

Once you have neutralized each of the experiences, then bring yourself back to the present time, open your eyes and come back to the present.

A variant of this exercise is to use a tape, such as the meditation binaural beat tape, and simply ask yourself in relaxed state, "What is the first experience in my life that led to this pattern?" Often that experience will pop into your mind briefly, and when it does, interact with it and provide information to yourself at that younger age in an emotionally clear and loving way to help let go of that hurt or pain. Also inquire as to what meaning you need from the event, and affirmatively note that you welcome the positive information and can let go of the unpleasant emotion.

What if a Past Life Pops Up?

If you ask yourself what the first experience of eating

problems was and you suddenly find yourself in another place or time, you may be experiencing a mental representation that would be typically referred to as a past-life experience.

It is important to realize that this experience neither proves nor disproves past lives in general, and you do not have to believe in past lives to have this experience. It can just be a means by which your mind is condensing the information to provide you with an answer to the question.

It could be a metaphorical experience, or it could be some form of conscious experience from a past life, either yours or someone else's, or tapping into a general aspect of the collective unconscious of feelings of deprivation or starvation or lack that you are touching into with your own consciousness through the experience.

There is no problem with this, and you deal with it in exactly the same way that you dealt with any of the other experiences; it is simply as if it were a past life. Treating it as if it is meaningful and therapeutic for yourself to do so will help it clear the pattern from your mind, whether it is from a past life or whether it is not from a past life.

I had the experience of performing this exercise on myself and receiving a sequence of experiences that would have appeared to be from past lives, typically from time periods where food was scarce. I interacted with each one of those experiences in a manner that was loving and caring and allowed that person to simply move on and thereby released a considerable amount of pressure towards eating in different contexts.

Again, I have no idea whether these were true past lives or whether these were mental representations that represented internal structure to me, but it really is irrelevant in the context of direct experience. Use these to your benefit irrespective of how you like to conceive of notions related to past lives.

BEHAVIOR TIP #9: WHEN YOU ORDER FOOD IN A RESTAURANT OR EVEN WHEN YOU LADLE FOOD OUT FOR YOURSELF AT HOME, EAT ANYTHING YOU LIKE BUT EAT EXACTLY HALF OF WHAT WAS SERVED.

This will not necessary work totally effectively if you are on a particular diet; however, halving your calorie intake will be of some use in weight loss irrespective.

I used to do this when I was in medical school, and I considered it the "poor student's diet" because after ordering one meal, you could easily make two or three meals out of it. It is, however, very easy to trick yourself when doing this into ordering a twelve-ounce steak instead of a six-ounce steak and eating half of the twelve-ounce steak, having the same amount of food you would have had had you ordered the six-ounce steak to start with, so you have to rigidly maintain the exact same ordering patterns when you go to restaurants that you would have were you not on the half-portion diet model.

This is an exceptionally difficult program to follow long term because it tends to evoke feelings of deprivation: *Why can*

I not eat it all? What is going on with this? However, it is a very interesting practice to try to see how successful you are at it and how long it will work, and as long as it does work, you can use it very effectively for weight loss.

Chapter Nineteen

Tap, Tap, Tapping

Emotional Freedom Technique

Gary Craig was an engineer who eventually decided that he would create a healing technique based upon the acupuncture points of the body, and he designed a technique called the Emotional Freedom Technique (EFT) which he has shared freely throughout the Internet. It is easy to Google "tapping points" and discover some of the sequences to be used in this technique. A recent review article of twenty-two research articles based upon tapping of acupuncture points found that each had statistically significant results in the positive direction. Whether the concept of the energy meridians is useful to you or whether you want to consider this as another means of getting past the gatekeeper is entirely your choice.

This is a unique series of techniques which works very differently than affirmations or hypnotic suggestions, and the reason for this is that rather than finding an affirmation that is ideal, the goal is to tap through the negative experience or the negative self-talk itself.

Some people are very uncomfortable with this if they have been working with affirmations for a long period of time because they believe speaking about something negatively will bring it into their lives, so some practitioners have modified the original EFT to do one round of negative followed by another round of positive. Gary is not in support of this modification at the date of this writing.

The original technique was designed to remove the negative unconscious suggestions that are floating around just outside of your awareness. Thus, you would tap on a sequence such as, "I hate myself because I'm overweight," or "I feel disgusted by my weight," or "I fail in my diet in every way" as the trigger sentence to go through with the purpose of removing the negative emotions attached.

Gary Craig's vision was since you are thinking this stuff anyway, you might as well deal with it consciously instead of pretending it is not there and trying to cover it with affirmations that do not work. Again, some have modified this technique to go through the first few sequences using the negative aspect, as I just described, and then following through with a follow-up that uses positive affirmations to presumably replace those negative feelings.

You can do as you see fit after exploring this interesting technique. What is striking about this model is that it follows a general principle that energy is the primary function and physicality follows. It is because you are changing energy systems by practicing this technique, which then eventually changes physical conditions.

I would be remiss if I did not share that when I first saw

this technique practiced my initial impression was that it had to be utterly ridiculous beyond words; however, I did suspend disbelief and practiced it a few times and found it to be amazingly powerful in spite of it not following traditional models or mechanisms that we would typically use in psychiatric practice. There is a growing following in these types of techniques under the general category of Energy Psychology.

I have seen DVDs, as an example, in which deeply traumatic experiences of wartime veterans were essentially eliminated in the course of twenty minutes, and it is hard to ignore observations like that.

How and Where to Tap

Without engaging in a long discussion of the reasons for each one of these points and the reasons for each one of these things, I will nevertheless describe it so that you can follow along in the experiences that will follow.

The first step is done in order to remove any psychological reversals. This is to tap what is called the "karate chop point," which is on the outer point of your hand, halfway between your wrist and the base of your pinky finger, and simply tap it constantly and make a statement, such as, "My weight is disgusting me. . ." Complete the sentence with, **"and I completely love and accept myself."**

Do that three times, and then you will continue tapping, just saying "weight:"

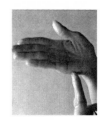

Tap at the edge of your eyebrow on the inside,

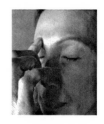

The outside of your eye,

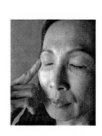

Underneath your eye in the center,

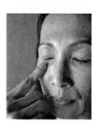

On top of your lip in the middle under your nose,

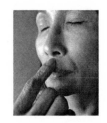

Under your lip,

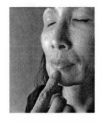

The spot under your clavicle in a soft spot about two inches from the center of your chest on either side,

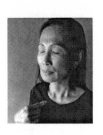

The soft spot on the side of your ribs roughly equivalent in height to the nipple line [men] or bra line [women],

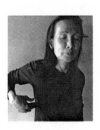

A spot at the bottom of your ribs two inches from the side at the bottom of your base rib [optional point],

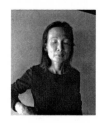

The top of your head [note: I like to end the sequence with this point, but Gary uses it first prior to the eyebrow point.].

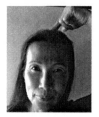

The way you will know you have identified these spots after looking at the diagrams is that virtually all of them feel tender to you. If you are tapping on a piece of skin, and it just feels like skin, you are not on the right spot. If you hit the spot and it feels tender on touch, that is the spot.

These are particular acupuncture points on traditional Chinese acupuncture lines. You will be activating many of the acupuncture meridians as you do this practice. The sequence as described is considered the basic sequence which is often all that is necessary using this model. Check links on the **www. newmindnewbody.com** website for the longer sequence for more challenging scenarios.

You can use this technique as I just described on any of the negative sentences, negative feelings, or negative experiences from any of the mind maps that you have completed up to this point, and I encourage you to do so; however, I am going to share two specific experiences now that you can use separately from the mind maps.

Be sure to ask yourself how true the negative feeling or statement is for you before you start any tapping sequence, and then repeat after the sequence. Use the first number that comes to mind. Notice the improvement. Repeat the sequence until the problem has cleared, which means that the number representing the "truth" of the statement should reduce to below two out of ten. If it hasn't, repeat the sequence until it does.

EXPERIENCE #24: TAP YOUR GOAL WEIGHT

First, ask yourself how true this sentence for you. Write down the first number from one to ten that comes to mind. Move on to your setup. Your setup sentence in this exercise is: *My perfect weight is* _____ *and I weigh* _____, *and I deeply love and completely accept myself.* The blank is the same number. For example, if you weigh 200 pounds and you are saying your goal weight is 150 pounds and your weight *is* 150 pounds, the immediate thing that will pop into your head is, "Who are you kidding? I weigh 200 pounds!" or "In a pig's eye!"

This is excellent! These statements are called "tailgaters," and they pop into your mind at unanticipated times during the exercise. It is very important to acknowledge the tailgaters and write them down. You are hoping to get tailgaters from these exercises; they are not to be avoided.

Tap on the karate point, my perfect goal weight is _____ and my weight is _____, and I deeply love and completely accept myself. Tap through the entire sequence of points simply saying, goal weight, the number; goal weight, the number, as you go through all of them. Repeat the sequence of points at least three times.

Ask yourself at the end how true you think this is of you. Take the first number that comes to mind. Compare it to the number before the tapping. Did it improve? If the number doesn't indicate a high degree of acceptance, then repeat the experience until it does.

Repeat this exercise daily for two weeks and follow what happens with your weight at the end of the two weeks. In addition, take those little tailgaters, writer them down and keep them available because we are going to deal with them in the next chapter.

EXPERIENCE #25: TAP IN FRONT OF THE MIRROR

This is an experience that will be deeply uncomfortable for some, yet it can also be extremely relieving if you persevere through it.

Strip naked in front of a full-length mirror and ask yourself how attractive you feel that you are on a one-to-ten scale. Accept the first number that comes to mind and write it down. If you have substantial issues with weight, your number will probably be very low. That is okay because you are going to transform this. Remember, hatred of your weight will tend to cause you to hold on to it because of emotional attachment.

Your setup statement is simply "I love and deeply accept myself." Just continue looking at the mirror and proceed through the tapping sequence over and over and over, and when you have gone through the tapping sequence about ten times, ask yourself the same question. Again, accept the first number that came to mind.

If it has gotten better by one or two numbers, that is fantastic, and probably represents a huge psychological change relating to you and your weight. Repeat the experience, keep tapping, and keep going through the points. Do not avert your gaze from the mirror. Keep looking at the mirror as you tap, and as you do, continue several more sequences through until you get at least four or five numbers' improvement in your ten-point scale.

You may not get this one all the way to a perfect number the first time through. That is okay. If you got four or five numbers' improvement, great! Repeat the experience in a few days and continue repeating it until you get an excellent, strong response that shows a positive perception of your body.

This will let go of the negative feelings that are helping you to hold on to the fact and by experiencing a sense of love and contentment with your body, it will help the fat go away. You will not have anything to hold on to, literally, emotionally, or soon enough, physically.

EXPERIENCE #26: TAP AND EAT

This is the last of the formal tapping exercises I am going to share; however, it is another means of dealing with food cravings to help them clear.

When you have an absolutely unbelievable craving for a particular food that you just cannot get rid of in any other way, go and grab a giant plate of that food and put it at the table in front of you and watch it and start to eat it and start going through this tapping exercise. Tap and tap and tap.

You will discover as you tap through the points while eating the craved food, the craving will begin to reduce. Continue tapping until the craving has reduced to one or zero on a numerical scale of one to ten.

T=Test — From Lead to Gold

Chapter Twenty

From Lead to Gold

Delicious Failure

Early on during your diet and in the initial period after your successful weight loss, there will be episodes where your newfound healthier eating patterns fail. This is an inevitable event in life, and it is deeply, deeply important to treasure these moments.

These are the interior lead that you can use in your own internal alchemy to change into gold. These can be the points of transformation. If everything to this point was relatively easy, that is awesome, but these are the final pieces that have to change for you to successfully complete your hero's journey. This is that last trial that is what really changes you as you change your eating.

Examples of these things occurring include the tailgating statements from your EFT practice. They include other things that pop out of your mind maps that have not been dealt with yet. They include the thoughts or the feelings that happen when you sit down in a new place and completely break every rule of your diet because something on the menu was calling to you so strongly you just could not say no.

Immediately – *immediately* – write this down. Write down what happened, the emotions that went along with it, and the experience and the location and the setting. Be aware of it, and first of all, let go of the negativity. This is an opportunity. It is not a failure by any standard.

Your unconscious has been changing throughout this process because you have been working on it using hypnotic scripts, using EFT practices, and using NLP techniques, and you have been dredging up more stuff, chopping out pearls, making new strings, but there still may be little remnants of stuff deep down there that has not yet changed, but it is much weaker than it ever was before, and it is clinging to its very existence. This is your chance to clean that last bit out.

Again, much as in the case of your fat itself in the parts experience, be grateful that little part made itself available to you to change rather than hiding away for longer where you would not even know it was there for another month or year. This gives you something to work on and gets you out of this final stuck point.

EXPERIENCE #27: IDENTIFY, DRAW, AND ASK

• When failure happens in whatever area that we just described relating to weight, identify the thought, feeling, place, person, or situation where you feel stuck, where things are not progressing or where you failed in a goal.

•Write down every detail that you can imagine as it comes to mind.

•If negative emotions arise, that is perfectly fine. Let them pass and do not hold on to them. Keep working at getting a detailed explanation.

•Now draw whatever this feeling is. It does not matter if you are an artist and it does not matter if it is nothing other than a big black blob on a piece of paper. It can be anything. It is not going to be judged and you are not going to frame it. Just draw it.

•Immediately after you draw it, look at it and ask it, "What are you trying to communicate to me that I have not yet heard? I truly want to know."

•Sit quietly and listen as you get some impression, thought, or idea as an answer to that question.

•Once you get that, look at the blob you have drawn and thank it for the information it has just shared with you. Mean it. From the bottom of your heart.

•Make that central point of information the core of a new mind map and draw out every potential branch from the mind map that you can think of that relates to emotions, feelings, ideas, associations, people, or things.

•Spend your time with this because this is a key piece of data that has made itself aware to you.

•Next, choose any of the previous exercises that are appropriate – the parts exercise, the EFT tapping, the NLP sequences, or self-hypnotic scripts – and work on this new issue that has arisen.

•This is a point of true transformation for you.

•If anything is left emotionally, use tapping to help clear out the last bit.

EXPERIENCE #28: WORK WITH WHAT ARISES

Often as you start through the above process from Exercise #27, yet more internal stuff will start to churn and arise. Sometimes spontaneous memories will appear or new interpretations of interactions with others or even new insights about yourself and your patterns.

This is awesome! It is more grist for the mill, more lead to turn into gold. Begin an inner dialog with any of these new things as they arise, write them down, and follow the same procedure. This is how you will transform your energetic string to hold new pearls, destroying that last bit of overdetermined aspects of the behavior.

**BEHAVIOR TIP #10: AVOID ALL ALCOHOL UNTIL
AT GOAL WEIGHT**

Alcohol has unique properties during the digestion process that will make losing weight more difficult than it needs to be. Choose to skip it for now, and know that you can enjoy it in reasonable portions once you achieve your goal weight.

T=Transform —— Long Term Success

Chapter Twenty-One

Success for the Long-Term

Hero – The New You

First, congratulate yourself as you have succeeded through what is truly an epic journey of losing weight.

Remember to use any setbacks that arise as yet another road to success and realize that although they are frustrating, they are a means as described in the previous chapter of further advancement. There may be a few missing pearls that eventually come to awareness later down the road, and that is okay because you have the skills, the knowledge, and the expertise to deal with them fully and clear them up completely.

One challenge, however, is to realize that once you are at your goal weight, you are able to eat a few additional calories each day, but it is not a free-for-all, so begin increasing calorie intake slowly, for example, by 100 calories per day, and make sure that you do not hit a point where weight gain returns.

If you slip five pounds over your goal weight, return to whatever diet was successful to you at the induction or the beginning most strict phase to get rid of those five pounds as quickly as possible. Again, realize if you have failed at a particular meal, it does not open the door to continuing to break the diet pattern. Use it as a onetime failure, learn from it, and return to the diet at the next meal.

New Frequency for Weight Checks

Because of the tendency to slide in your diet after the diet is "over," there is a tendency for weight to come back. Remember that underlying fantasy that all of us have that we can eat whatever we want now and remain at our lower weight. That may continue to operate at some level, so weigh at least weekly for the first year after successful weight loss.

This is a more frequent weighing than during the actual weight loss period, and the reason is that we need to monitor the weight more carefully now so that it does not creep up in between weigh-ins due to us being a little bit too lax in our diet.

Think back to one of the first experiences, which was choosing the diet right for you based upon diet plans. If you did this, made some minor food substitutions and dealt with the sense of deprivation, you really should not feel like you are on a diet right now; you should feel like you are eating the food that you want to eat for the rest of your life; thus, breaking out of the general pattern you have established should not be seen as an emotionally driven act. I am still shocked that I enjoy broccoli and cauliflower now to the degree that I actually miss it when I do not have either for just a few days. This is a truly new me.

If it does become an emotionally driven act, go back to

the previous chapter and run through the sequence to find out why.

EXPERIENCE #29: YOU ARE THE HERO, AND YOU HAVE FINISHED THE SEQUENCE OF JOSEPH CAMPBELL'S HERO CYCLE.

You have, in fact, accepted the call to adventure. You have overcome the minor obstacles that usually act as a guardian and deterrent to keep you from your goal, and you have also mastered the massive final conflict of dealing with those parts of yourself that were not in alignment with your conscious wishes.

Now is the time to finalize that fourth stage of the hero's journey, that is, to come back and solidify and ground this experience in your world to make it real and to make it last, so this experience is to write your story of weight loss in this sequence of the hero's journey and to describe it in exquisite detail for yourself.

Describe what called you to action, what called you to adventure, what led you to actually decide to succeed this time, then describe each of the personal challenges you met as you dealt with the internal conflict between your unconscious desire and your conscious plan, and finally, describe in as much detail as comfortable those areas of yourself that made deep internal change so that dieting is no longer a diet, but dieting is simply an ongoing lifestyle.

Finally, write down the final sequence, which is how you are going to bring this back to the world to share with others or to speak with others about it.

Congratulate yourself. You are a success!

Ten Behavior Tips

Experiences

CPSIA information can be obtained at www.ICGtesting.com
Printed in the USA
BVOW02s0508100715

408018BV00001B/135/P